Grow To Heal

A Guide to cultivating Medicinal Herbs and using their Transformative Power

Richard Myers & Shawn Joseph

Stay Loyal to the Soil

— FARMER SHAWN
HAPPY GROWING

Copyright © 2023 - All rights reserved.

The content contained within this book may not be reproduced, duplicated, or transmitted without direct written permission from the author or the publisher.

Under no circumstances will any blame or legal responsibility be held against the publisher, or author, for any damages, reparation, or monetary loss due to the information contained within this book. Either directly or indirectly.

Legal Notice:

This book is copyright protected. This book is only for personal use. You cannot amend, distribute, sell, use, quote, or paraphrase any part, or the content within this book, without the consent of the author or publisher.

Disclaimer Notice:

Please note the information contained within this document is for educational and entertainment purposes only. All effort has been executed to present accurate, up-to-date, and reliable, complete information. No warranties of any kind are declared or implied. Readers acknowledge that the author is not engaging in the rendering of legal, financial, medical, or professional advice. The content within this book has been derived from various sources. Please consult a licensed professional before attempting any techniques outlined in this book.

By reading this document, the reader agrees that under no circumstances is the author responsible for any losses, direct or indirect, which are incurred as a result of the use of the information contained within this document, including, but not limited to, — errors, omissions, or inaccuracies.

ISBN:

Summary:

In this book, we embark on a journey that invites you to become a steward of your own well-being by cultivating medicinal herbs in your own home or garden. By learning the art of growing these remarkable plants, you will not only nurture their growth but also nurture a deeper connection to the healing power of nature, learning how these botanical treasures can support our physical, mental, and emotional well-being.

Within these pages, we will explore the practical aspects of growing medicinal herbs, sharing the history of each plant, recipes for the use of each herb and much more. You will discover that regardless of your level of gardening experience, you can create an abundant oasis of healing plants, fostering an environment that harmonizes with the cycles of nature and fosters your own well-being while harnessing the potential of these extraordinary plants.

With each turn, you will not only learn how to grow a diverse array of medicinal herbs, each with its unique story, characteristics, and therapeutic benefits. You will also discover how recipes with chamomile can calm a restless mind, how potent ginseng tincture can invigorate weary souls, and how to make lavender tea that will lull you into peaceful slumber. Uncover the secrets of versatile plants like turmeric, echinacea, and maca root, which offer a multitude of health-enhancing properties.

Table of Contents:

Introduction i
    Quotes ii

Why Should One Attempt to Gain Knowledge About Natural Medicine? 1
    Why Would Someone Use Medicinal Drugs? 3
    What Is The History Of Medicinal Plants 4

Broadleaf Plantain 7
    History of Broadleaf Plantain 8
    How to Grow Broadleaf Plantain 8
    How to Clone Broadleaf Plantain 9
    How is Broadleaf Plantain Medicinal 9
    Medicinal Recipes for Broadleaf Plantain: 10

Chamomile 13
    History of Chamomile 14
    How to Grow Chamomile 14
    How to Clone Chamomile 15
    How to Divide Chamomile 16
    How is Chamomile Medicinal 16
    Medicinal Chamomile Recipes 17

Cleavers (Galium aparine) 19
    History of Galium Aparine 20
    How to Grow Cleaver Plant 20
    How to Clone Galium Aparine Plant 21
    How is Galium Aparine Medicinal 22
    Medicinal Cleaver Recipes 22

Dandelion 25
History of Dandelion 26
How to Grow Dandelion 26
How to Clone Dandelion Plants 27
How is Dandelion Medicinal 28
Medicinal Recipes with Dandelion 29

Dong Quai 31
History of Dong Quai 32
How to Grow Dong Quai 32
How to Clone Dong Quai 33
How is Dong Quai Medicinal 34
Medicinal Recipes for Dong Quai 35

Echinacea 37
History of Echinacea 38
How to Grow Echinacea 38
How to Clone Echinacea 39
How is Echinacea Medicinal 40
Medicinal Echinacea Recipes 41

Feverfew 43
History of Feverfew Plant 44
How to Grow Feverfew 44
How to Clone Feverfew Plant 45
How is Feverfew Medicinal 45
Medicinal Feverfew Recipes 46

Ginger 47
History of Ginger 48
How to Grow Ginger 48
Can You Clone Ginger? 49
How is Ginger Medicinal? 50
Medicinal Ginger Recipe 50

Gingko 53
History of Ginkgo Plant 54
How to Grow Gingko 54
How to Clone Ginkgo Plant 55
How is Ginkgo Plant Medicinal 55
Medicinal Ginkgo Recipes 56

Ginseng 57
History of Ginseng 58
How to Grow Ginseng 58
How to Clone Ginseng 59
How is Ginseng Medicinal 59
Medicinal Ginseng Recipes 60

Goldenseal 61
History of Goldenseal 62
How to Grow Goldenseal 62
How to Clone Goldenseal 63
How is Goldenseal Medicinal 63
Medicinal Goldenseal Recipes 64

Holy Basil 65
History of Holy Basil 66
How to Grow Holy Basil 66
How to Clone Holy Basil Tulsi Plant 67
How is Holy Basil Medicinal 68
Medicinal Recipes for Holy Basil 69

Lavender 71
History of Lavender Plant 72
How to Grow Lavender 72
How to Clone Lavender Plant 73
How is Lavender Medicinal 74
Medicinal Recipes with Lavender 75

Lemongrass 77
History of Lemongrass 78
How to Grow Lemongrass 78
How is Lemongrass Medicinal 79
Medicinal Lemongrass Recipes 79

Rosemary 81
History of Rosemary Plant 82
How to Grow Rosemary 82
How to Clone Rosemary Plant 83
How is Rosemary Medicinal 84
Medicinal Recipes with Rosemary 84

Sage 87
History of Sage Plant 88
How to Grow Sage 88
How to Clone Sage Plant 89
How is Sage Medicinal 90
Medicinal Recipes with Sage 90

Saint John's Wort 93
History of Saint John's Wort 94
How to Grow Saint John's Wort 94
How to Clone Saint John's Wort 95
How is Saint John's Wort Medicinal 95
Medicinal Saint John's Wort Recipes 96

Valerian Root 97
History of Valerian Plant 98
How to Grow Valerian Root 98
How to Clone Valerian 99
How is Valerian Medicinal 99
Medicinal Valerian Recipes 100

Witch Hazel 103
    History of Witch Hazel 104
    How to Grow Witch Hazel 104
    How to Clone Witch Hazel 105
    How is Witch Hazel Medicinal? 105
    Medicinal Witch Hazel Recipes 106

Infections & Medicinal Plants That May Help 108

Medicinal Plants Found in the USA 111

Medicinal Plants Specifically for Men 115

Medicinal Plants Specifically for Women 118

Endangered Medicinal Plants: (Found in North America) 122

About Authors 125

Introduction

In a world driven by technological advancements and modern medicine, it's easy to overlook the remarkable healing properties found within the embrace of nature. For centuries, civilizations across the globe have turned to medicinal herbs as their trusted allies in the pursuit of health and well-being. These miraculous plants, gifted to us by Mother Earth have served as invaluable sources of relief, rejuvenation, and profound healing. What if we told you that the key to unlocking vitality and promoting holistic wellness could be found right in your backyard or windowsill? Welcome to "Grow To Heal : A Guide to cultivating Medicinal Herbs and using their Transformative Power.

In this book, we go on a journey that invites you to become a steward of your own well-being by cultivating medicinal herbs in your own home or garden. By learning the art of growing these remarkable plants, you will not only nurture their growth but also nurture a deeper connection to the healing power of nature, learning how these botanical treasures can support our physical, mental, and emotional well-being.

Within these pages, we will explore the practical aspects of growing medicinal herbs, sharing the history of each plant, recipes for the use of each herb and much more. You will discover that regardless of your level of gardening experience, you can create an abundant oasis of healing plants, fostering an environment that harmonizes with the cycles of nature and fosters your own well-being while harnessing the potential of these extraordinary plants.

With each turn, you will not only learn how to grow a diverse array of medicinal herbs, each with its unique story, characteristics, and therapeutic benefits. You will also discover how recipes with chamomile can calm a restless mind, how potent ginseng tincture can invigorate weary souls, and how to make lavender tea that will lull you into peaceful slumber. Uncover the secrets of versatile plants like turmeric, echinacea, and maca root, which offer a multitude of health-enhancing properties.

But growing medicinal herbs is not just about acquiring knowledge—it is a transformative journey that invites you to slow down, engage your senses, and embrace the profound healing connection between plants and humans. Alongside the practical guidance, you will get the history of each plant as well as their medicinal use that will deepen your relationship with the natural world.

Whether you're a seasoned herbal enthusiast with a sprawling garden or just beginning your journey with a cozy balcony, "Grow To Heal" will be your trusted companion, providing insights, practical recipes, and growing tips. Step into this world where the fragrance of herbs dances in the air, where the gentle touch of a leaf can spark profound transformation, and where the rhythm of nature's heartbeat resonates within us all.

So, let us set out on this journey together—a journey of growth, knowledge, connection, and health. With your hands in the soil and your heart aligned with the wisdom of nature, you will uncover the profound rewards of growing medicinal herbs, both for your garden and your own well-being creating a harmonious coexistence with the extraordinary world of medicinal herbs. Get ready to open your heart, embrace the wisdom of Mother Earth, and prepare to be amazed by the transformative power of these remarkable botanical allies.

Quotes

The herbs are for the healing of the nations. - **Revelation 22:2**

God gives us the use of plants and herbs for curative care, both physical - **2 Kings 20:7; Psalm 51:7**

"There are no worthless herbs — only the lack of knowledge." - **Avicenna**

"Every green herb, from the lotus to the darnel, is rich with delicate aids to help incurious man." - **Martin Farquhar Tupper**

"Much Virtue in Herbs, little in Men." - **Benjamin Franklin**

"Out of 40,000+ herbs used worldwide, perhaps only 50-60 of them are tonic superherbs. These superherbs should be taken for long periods, because, like all tonics, they are more like food and they build health treasures within and nourish our "stress defense shield." - **David Wolfe**

....

Why Should One Attempt to Gain Knowledge About Natural Medicine?

1. Holistic Approach: Natural medicine often takes a holistic approach to health and well-being, considering the interconnectedness of the body, mind, and spirit. It aims to address the root causes of health issues rather than just alleviating symptoms.

2. Minimal Side Effects: Natural remedies, such as herbal supplements, are generally perceived to have fewer side effects compared to pharmaceutical drugs. Many people prefer the idea of using substances that occur naturally in nature rather than synthetic chemicals.

3. Cultural and Traditional Practices: Natural medicine has a long history in many cultures, and people often rely on traditional remedies that have been passed down through generations. Traditional systems like Ayurveda, Traditional Chinese Medicine (TCM), and Indigenous healing practices incorporate natural remedies as a central part of their healthcare systems.

4. Personal Beliefs and Values: Some individuals may have personal beliefs or values that align with natural medicine. They may prefer a more natural and non-invasive approach to healing, promoting the body's innate ability to heal itself.

5. Complementary and Integrative Medicine: Natural medicine is often used alongside conventional medicine as a complementary or integrative approach. Many people seek natural remedies to supplement their conventional treatments, aiming to enhance overall health and well-being.

6. Environmental Concerns: Some individuals choose natural medicine out of environmental considerations. They may prefer products that are sustainably sourced, organic, and do not contribute to the pollution or depletion of natural resources.

7. Historical use and knowledge: Natural drugs have been used for their therapeutic properties for centuries. Plants and other natural substances have been utilized for their healing effects, pain relief, and psychoactive properties. Traditional medicine systems such as Ayurveda, Traditional Chinese Medicine, and indigenous healing practices have relied on natural drugs.

8. Availability and accessibility: Natural drugs are often readily available and accessible in various regions. Plants and fungi containing psychoactive compounds, such as marijuana, psilocybin mushrooms, and coca leaves, have been traditionally used in specific areas where they naturally occur.

9. Desire for alternative treatments: Some people turn to natural drugs as an alternative to conventional medicine or pharmaceutical drugs. They may seek out natural remedies for various health conditions or simply prefer a more holistic approach to their well-being.

10. Perception of safety and reduced side effects: Natural drugs are often perceived as safer or having fewer side effects compared to synthetic drugs. While this is not always the case, the belief that natural substances are inherently safer can influence people's decisions to use them.

11. Curiosity and exploration: Humans have a natural inclination to explore altered states of consciousness and seek novel experiences. Natural drugs can provide unique psychoactive effects, leading individuals to experiment with them out of curiosity or for recreational purposes.

12. Changing societal attitudes: In recent years, there has been a growing acceptance and interest in exploring the potential benefits of natural drugs. Research into the therapeutic use of substances like psilocybin, MDMA, and cannabis has gained momentum, leading to increased discussions about their potential positive impacts.

Why Would Someone Use Medicinal Drugs?

- People use medicinal drugs for several reasons, primarily to treat and manage various health conditions. Here are some common motivations:

1. Treating Illnesses: Medicinal drugs are designed to target specific diseases, infections, or health conditions. They are formulated to alleviate symptoms, cure diseases, or manage chronic conditions, aiming to restore or improve health.

2. Medical Recommendations: Healthcare professionals, such as doctors, prescribe medicinal drugs based on their expertise and knowledge of a patient's medical condition. People trust the advice of medical professionals and rely on prescribed drugs to address their health concerns.

3. Scientifically Proven Efficacy: Medicinal drugs undergo rigorous testing and clinical trials to determine their safety and effectiveness. People trust that these drugs have been thoroughly evaluated and approved by regulatory authorities, such as the Food and Drug Administration (FDA) in the United States or the European Medicines Agency (EMA) in Europe.

4. Symptom Relief: Medicinal drugs often provide quick relief from symptoms associated with various health conditions. They can alleviate pain, reduce inflammation, suppress coughs, lower fevers, and offer other symptomatic relief.

5. Managing Chronic Conditions: Many individuals with chronic illnesses, such as diabetes, hypertension, or autoimmune diseases, rely on medicinal drugs to manage their conditions and maintain their health. These drugs help control symptoms, prevent complications, and improve quality of life.

6. Life-Saving Interventions: In some cases, medicinal drugs are essential for saving lives. For instance, emergency medications, such as epinephrine for severe allergic reactions or anticoagulants for preventing blood clots, are crucial in critical situations.

7. Advanced Medical Treatments: Medicinal drugs are often integral to advanced medical treatments, such as chemotherapy for cancer or immunosuppressants for organ transplant recipients. These drugs play a critical role in combating diseases and supporting complex medical procedures.

What Is The History Of Medicinal Plants

The use of medicinal plants dates back thousands of years and is intertwined with the history of human civilization. Here is a brief overview of the history of medicinal plants.

Ancient Times:

Prehistoric Evidence: Archaeological findings suggest that early humans used plants for medicinal purposes. Fossilized remains of medicinal plants, such as yarrow and marshmallow, have been found at Neanderthal burial sites dating back over 60,000 years.

Ancient Civilizations: Ancient civilizations, including the Sumerians, Egyptians, Chinese, and Indians, developed sophisticated systems of herbal medicine. They documented the medicinal properties of various plants and incorporated them into their healing practices. For example, the Ebers Papyrus from ancient Egypt, dating back to around 1550 BCE, contains detailed information on medicinal plants and their uses.

Classical Era:

Greek and Roman Influence: Greek physicians, such as Hippocrates (known as the "Father of Medicine") and Dioscorides, made significant contributions to herbal medicine. Hippocrates emphasized the healing power of nature and used medicinal plants in his treatments. Dioscorides compiled a comprehensive book called "De Materia Medica," which described over 600 plants and their therapeutic properties. The Romans, influenced by Greek knowledge, continued to explore and use medicinal plants.

Medieval Period:

Arab and Islamic Contributions: During the medieval period, Islamic scholars played a vital role in preserving and expanding the knowledge of medicinal plants. The works of physicians like Avicenna (Ibn Sina) and Al-Razi (Rhazes) became influential in the field of herbal medicine. They compiled comprehensive texts on herbal remedies and classification systems.

European Herbalism: In Europe, herbal medicine continued to be practiced and evolved during the Middle Ages. Monastic gardens were established, cultivating and studying medicinal plants. Prominent herbalists, such as Hildegard von Bingen and Paracelsus, made notable contributions to herbal medicine during this period.

Modern Era:

Scientific Advancements: The 18th and 19th centuries saw significant developments in pharmacology and chemistry. Scientists began isolating and synthesizing active compounds from medicinal plants, leading to the discovery of important drugs. For example, the discovery of salicylic acid from willow bark led to the development of aspirin.

Traditional Medicine Systems: Traditional medicine systems, such as Ayurveda, Traditional Chinese Medicine (TCM), and Indigenous healing practices, continued to flourish and were recognized for their contributions to healthcare. These systems utilize numerous medicinal plants and herbal remedies as part of their holistic approaches.

Modern Pharmaceutical Industry: The 20th century witnessed the rise of the modern pharmaceutical industry, with a focus on synthetic drugs. However, even today, many pharmaceutical drugs are derived from or inspired by natural compounds found in plants.

Throughout history, the use of medicinal plants has played a crucial role in healthcare and has contributed to the development of modern medicine. Today, traditional herbal medicine and the scientific exploration of plant-derived compounds continue to coexist and offer diverse options for healthcare and well-being.

Broadleaf Plantain

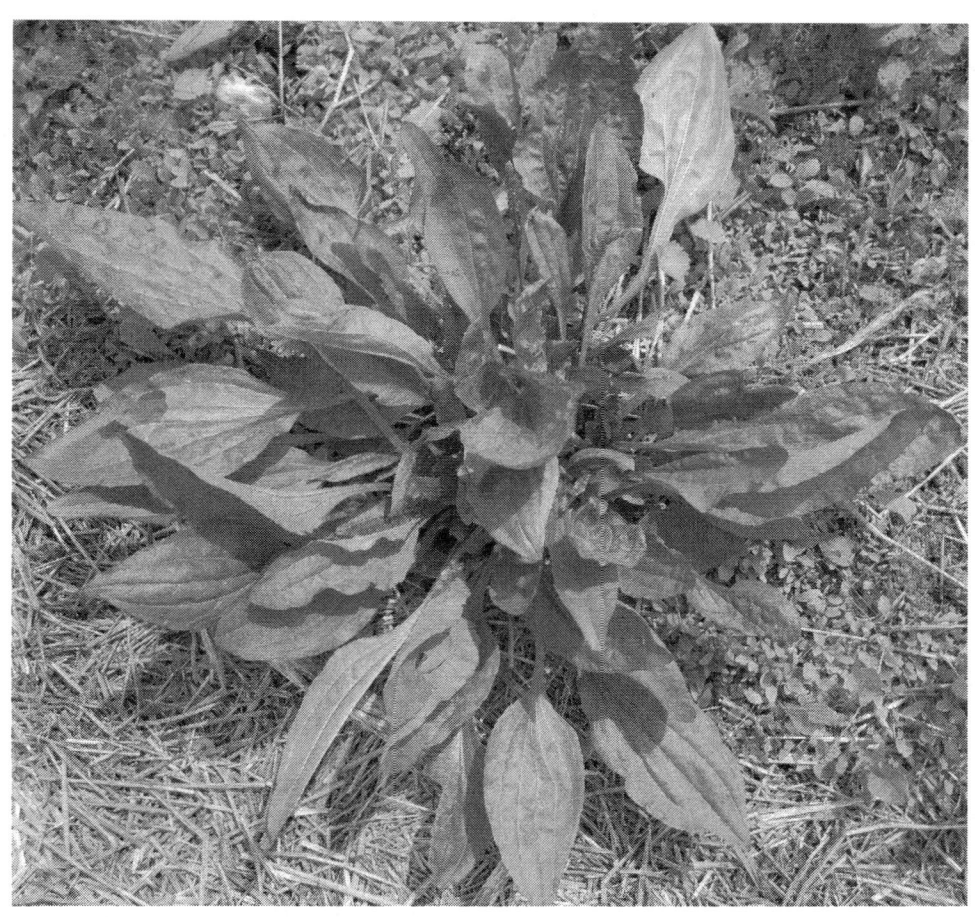

History of Broadleaf Plantain

Broadleaf plantain, also known as Plantago major, is a common weed that is found in many parts of the world. It has a long history of use in traditional medicine and has been used for its medicinal properties for thousands of years.

Broadleaf plantain is native to Europe and Asia, but it has been naturalized in many other parts of the world, including North America, where it was introduced by European settlers in the 17th century. It is now found in almost every region of the world.

The plant has been used for medicinal purposes for centuries. The ancient Greeks used it to treat wounds, and it was also used in traditional Chinese medicine to treat a variety of ailments. Native Americans used it for many purposes, including as a poultice for wounds, as a tea for digestive issues, and as a treatment for fever.

During the Middle Ages, broadleaf plantain was considered to be a "cure-all" and was used to treat a wide variety of ailments, including respiratory infections, digestive issues, and skin conditions. It was also used as a pain reliever and as a remedy for insect bites and stings.

Today, broadleaf plantain is still used for its medicinal properties and is often found in herbal remedies and natural health products. It is used to treat a variety of conditions, including digestive issues, respiratory infections, and skin conditions. It is also used as a natural remedy for insect bites and stings, and as a pain reliever.

How to Grow Broadleaf Plantain

Broadleaf plantain, also known as Plantago major, is a hardy, easy-to-grow herb that can thrive in a variety of growing conditions. Here are the steps to grow broadleaf plantain:

Choose a suitable location: Broadleaf plantain can grow in full sun to partial shade and in a range of soil types, but prefers moist, well-drained soil with plenty of organic matter.

Prepare the soil: Broadleaf plantain grows well in soil that has been amended with compost or other organic matter. Loosen the soil to a depth of 6 to 8 inches and remove any rocks or debris.

Plant the seeds: Broadleaf plantain can be grown from seed. Sow the seeds directly in the garden soil in the spring, after the last frost, or in the fall. Plant the seeds about 1/4 inch deep and 6 inches apart.

Water and fertilize: Keep the soil moist but not waterlogged, especially during the plant's early growth stages. Fertilize with a balanced organic fertilizer every 4-6 weeks.

Control weeds: Broadleaf plantain can be invasive, so be sure to control weeds in the area where it is growing. Hand pulling or hoeing can be effective methods of weed control.

Harvest the leaves: Broadleaf plantain leaves can be harvested as soon as they are large enough to use, typically in early summer. The leaves can be used fresh or dried for later use.

Broadleaf plantain is a hardy plant that does not require much maintenance, making it an ideal choice for novice gardeners.

How to Clone Broadleaf Plantain

Broadleaf plantain can be easily propagated through seed or by dividing an established plant. Here are the steps to clone broadleaf plantain through division:

Choose a healthy broadleaf plantain plant and dig it up carefully, making sure to preserve as much of the root system as possible.

Use a sharp, clean knife to cut the root system into several pieces. Each piece should have at least one healthy shoot and a good portion of root. Plant the divided pieces into pots or directly into the garden soil. Make sure the soil is well-draining and rich in organic matter.

Water the newly planted divisions thoroughly and keep the soil moist but not waterlogged.

Keep the newly planted divisions in a shaded area for a few days to help them establish roots before exposing them to full sun.

Once the divisions have established roots and new growth, they can be transplanted to their permanent location in the garden.

Propagation through division is best done in the spring or fall when the plant is actively growing.

How is Broadleaf Plantain Medicinal

Broadleaf plantain, also known as Plantago major, is used for its medicinal properties. The plant contains a number of beneficial compounds, including allantoin, aucubin, and mucilage, which give it its healing properties.

Here are some ways in which broadleaf plantain is used medicinally:

Wound Healing: Broadleaf plantain is commonly used to promote wound healing. The allantoin in the plant helps to stimulate the growth of new skin cells, while the mucilage helps to soothe and moisturize the skin.

Digestive Health: Broadleaf plantain is used to promote digestive health. It has anti-inflammatory properties that can help to soothe inflamed digestive tissues. It also has a mild laxative effect and can help to relieve constipation.

Respiratory Health: Broadleaf plantain can be used to support respiratory health. It has expectorant properties that can help to loosen and expel phlegm from the lungs. It also has anti-inflammatory properties that can help to soothe inflamed respiratory tissues.

Skin Health: Broadleaf plantain can be used to promote skin health. The plant contains compounds that have antibacterial and anti-inflammatory properties, which can help to soothe and heal skin irritations such as rashes, eczema, and psoriasis.

Pain Relief: Broadleaf plantain can be used as a natural pain reliever. The plant contains compounds that have analgesic properties and can help to reduce pain and inflammation in the body.

Broadleaf plantain can be consumed as a tea, tincture, or used externally as a poultice or ointment. It can also be found in many herbal remedies and natural health products.

Medicinal Recipes for Broadleaf Plantain:

Broadleaf Plantain Tea: To make a tea, steep 1-2 teaspoons of dried broadleaf plantain leaves in a cup of hot water for 5-10 minutes. Strain and drink up to 3 cups per day. This tea can help soothe the digestive system, promote respiratory health, and support wound healing.

Broadleaf plantain salve:

Ingredients:

- 1 cup of broadleaf plantain leaves (fresh or dried)
- 1 cup of carrier oil (such as olive oil, coconut oil, or almond oil)
- 1 ounce of beeswax (grated or in pellet form)
- Optional: a few drops of essential oil for fragrance (e.g., lavender, tea tree)

Instructions:

1. If using fresh broadleaf plantain leaves, wash them thoroughly and pat dry. If using dried leaves, skip this step.

2. Chop the broadleaf plantain leaves into smaller pieces to release their properties.

3. In a heatproof jar or double boiler, combine the chopped broadleaf plantain leaves and the carrier oil.

4. Gently heat the mixture over low heat, either using a double boiler or by placing the jar in a pot of simmering water.

5. Let the mixture infuse for 1-2 hours, stirring occasionally. Ensure the oil doesn't get too hot or start boiling.

6. After infusing, remove the jar from heat and strain the oil through a fine-mesh sieve or cheesecloth into a clean bowl.

7. Return the strained oil to the heatproof jar or double boiler and add the grated beeswax.

8. Heat the mixture again over low heat until the beeswax is fully melted and combined with the oil.

9. If desired, add a few drops of essential oil for fragrance and stir well.

10. Carefully pour the mixture into clean, sterilized jars or tins.

11. Allow the salve to cool and solidify completely before sealing the containers.

12. Label and store the broadleaf plantain salve in a cool, dry place.

To use the salve, simply apply a small amount to the affected area of the skin as needed. Broadleaf plantain salve is commonly used for soothing skin irritations, insect bites, minor cuts, and other skin issues. However, it's always a good idea to perform a patch test on a small area of skin before using any new product, especially if you have known allergies or sensitivities.

Broadleaf plantain poultice:

Ingredients:

- Fresh broadleaf plantain leaves (enough to cover the affected area)
- Warm water (as needed)

Instructions:

1. Harvest fresh broadleaf plantain leaves from a clean and pesticide-free area.
2. Wash the leaves thoroughly to remove any dirt or debris.
3. Take a few leaves and gently crush them using a mortar and pestle or by rolling a clean glass or rolling pin over them. Crushing the leaves helps release their healing compounds.
4. Place the crushed leaves directly onto the affected area. If the area is too large, you can layer the leaves to cover it entirely.
5. Secure the poultice in place using a clean cloth or medical gauze.
6. If the leaves are not adhering well or if you prefer a moist poultice, you can dampen the leaves with warm water before applying them to the skin.
7. Leave the poultice on for 15-30 minutes or as needed.
8. Remove the poultice and discard the used plantain leaves.
9. Gently clean the area with warm water and pat it dry.
10. You can repeat the process multiple times a day if desired, replacing the poultice with fresh broadleaf plantain leaves each time.

Broadleaf plantain poultices are commonly used for their soothing and healing properties on skin irritations, insect bites, minor cuts, burns, and other skin issues. However, if you have known allergies or sensitivities, it's always a good idea to perform a patch test on a small area of skin before applying the poultice. Additionally, consult with a healthcare professional for persistent or severe skin conditions.

Chamomile

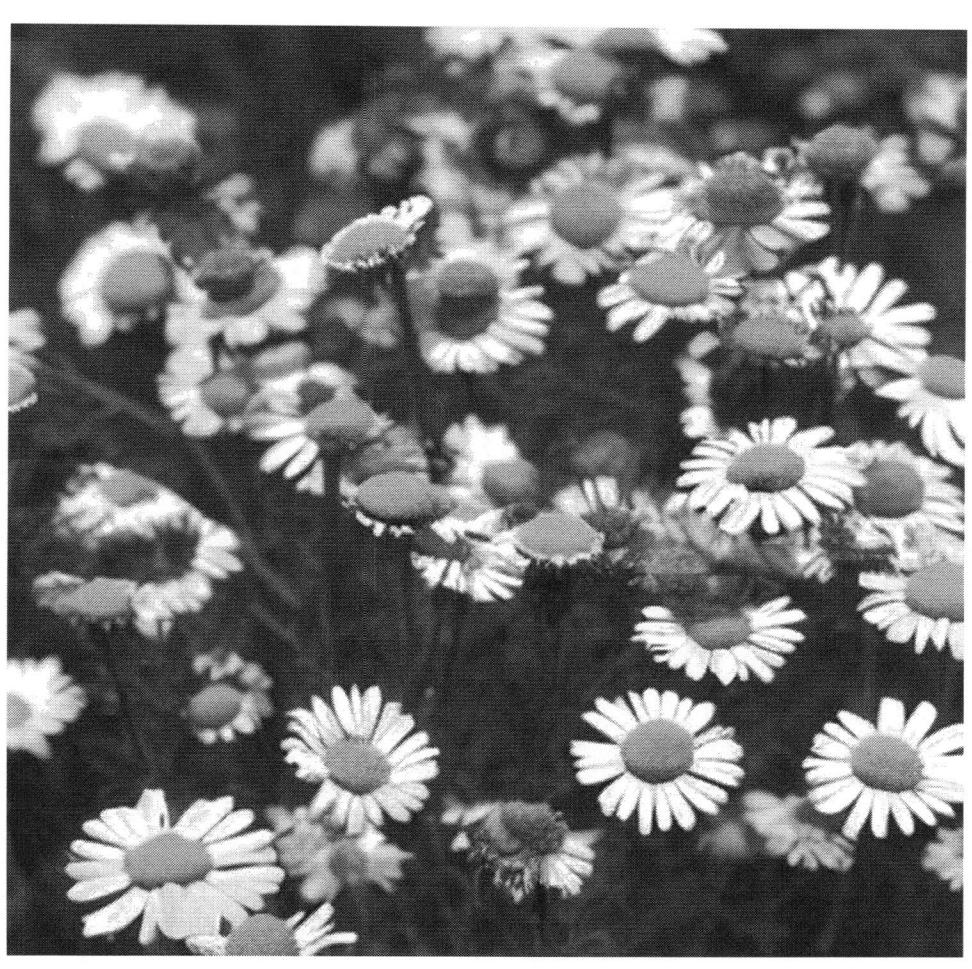

History of Chamomile

Chamomile has a long and rich history of use as a medicinal herb, dating back thousands of years to ancient Egypt, Greece, and Rome. The name "chamomile" is derived from the Greek words "chamai" and "melos," which mean "ground" and "apple," respectively, referring to the plant's low-growing habit and its apple-like scent.

In ancient Egypt, chamomile was used as a remedy for fever and as a cosmetic, and was also considered a sacred herb. It was dedicated to the sun god Ra, and was used in the embalming process to help preserve the bodies of the deceased.

In ancient Greece, chamomile was used as a remedy for a variety of ailments, including fever, inflammation, and nervousness. It was also used as a cosmetic, and was said to have been a favorite of Cleopatra.

In ancient Rome, chamomile was used as a remedy for digestive issues, and was also used in bathes and as a cosmetic.

Chamomile continued to be used throughout the Middle Ages and into the Renaissance, and was introduced to North America by European settlers in the 16th century.

Today, chamomile is still widely used for its medicinal properties, particularly for its calming and relaxing effects. It is commonly used in teas, as well as in tinctures, essential oils, and other herbal remedies.

How to Grow Chamomile

Chamomile is a relatively easy herb to grow, and it can thrive in a variety of climates. Here are some steps for growing chamomile:

Choose a location: Chamomile prefers full sun but can also grow in partial shade. It needs well-draining soil and does best in soil that is slightly acidic with a pH of 5.6-7.5.

Start from seeds or plants: Chamomile can be grown from seeds or transplants. If starting from seeds, plant them in the spring or fall, directly in the ground or in containers. The seeds should be planted shallowly, just beneath the soil surface. If using transplants, plant them in the ground or containers at the same depth as they were in their original pots.

Water regularly: Chamomile needs regular watering, especially during hot, dry weather. However, it is important not to overwater, as this can lead to root rot.

Fertilize occasionally: Chamomile does not require much fertilizer, but you can give it a boost by adding compost or a balanced fertilizer to the soil in the spring.

Harvest the flowers: Chamomile flowers can be harvested once they are fully open, which usually occurs in mid to late summer. Pinch the flowers off the stem and dry them for later use in tea or other remedies.

Allow the plant to self-seed: Chamomile is an annual plant, but it can self-seed and come back year after year. Allow the flowers to dry and go to seed, and they will drop and produce new plants the following year.

By following these steps, you should be able to grow healthy chamomile plants that produce an abundance of flowers for use in teas, salves, and other medicinal remedies.

How to Clone Chamomile

Chamomile can be propagated by division or by taking stem cuttings. Here are the steps for cloning chamomile using stem cuttings:

Choose a healthy plant: Select a chamomile plant that is healthy and disease-free to take cuttings from. Make sure the plant has plenty of new growth.

Take stem cuttings: Using clean, sharp scissors or pruning shears, take 3-4 inch cuttings from the new growth of the plant. Make the cut just below a leaf node.

Remove lower leaves: Remove the lower leaves from the stem cutting, leaving only a few leaves near the top of the cutting.

Dip in rooting hormone: Dip the bottom of the cutting in rooting hormone to encourage root growth.

Plant the cutting: Plant the cutting in a pot filled with a mixture of potting soil and perlite. Make sure the cutting is planted deep enough that the remaining leaves are above the soil surface.

Water and care for the cutting: Water the cutting thoroughly and place it in a warm, bright location out of direct sunlight. Keep the soil moist but not waterlogged, and mist the cutting daily to maintain humidity.

Transplant the cutting: Once the cutting has developed roots, which can take several weeks, transplant it into a larger pot or directly into the ground in a location with well-draining soil and full sun.

By following these steps, you should be able to successfully clone your chamomile plant and produce a new, healthy plant for use in teas, salves, and other remedies.

How to Divide Chamomile

Dividing chamomile is another way to propagate the plant and increase your chamomile stock. Here are the steps for dividing chamomile:

Choose the right time: The best time to divide chamomile is in the spring or fall, when the plant is not actively blooming.

Lift the plant: Carefully dig up the chamomile plant, trying not to damage the roots. You can use a garden fork or hand trowel to do this.

Separate the root ball: Once you have lifted the plant, gently separate the root ball into smaller sections using your hands or a clean garden knife. Each section should have some roots and healthy top growth.

Replant: Replant each section in a new location, spacing them about 8-12 inches apart. Make sure the soil is well-draining and the plants receive plenty of sunlight.

Water and care for the plants: Water the newly transplanted chamomile plants thoroughly, and keep the soil moist but not waterlogged. Chamomile does not require a lot of fertilizer, but you can add compost or a balanced fertilizer to the soil to give the plants a boost.

By following these steps, you should be able to successfully divide your chamomile plant and produce new, healthy plants for use in teas, salves, and other remedies.

How is Chamomile Medicinal

Chamomile is a medicinal herb that has been used for centuries to treat a wide range of ailments. It is believed to have a calming and relaxing effect on the body and mind, and is often used as a natural remedy for anxiety, insomnia, and stress.

Chamomile is also known for its anti-inflammatory and antioxidant properties. It contains a compound called chamazulene, which is believed to help reduce inflammation in the body and relieve pain. Chamomile is often used to treat digestive issues such as gas, bloating, and stomach cramps, as well as to relieve menstrual cramps.

Other potential health benefits of chamomile include its ability to boost the immune system, improve skin health, and reduce symptoms of allergies and asthma. Chamomile is also used topically to treat skin conditions such as eczema, psoriasis, and minor wounds.

Chamomile is most commonly consumed as a tea, but it can also be found in tinctures, capsules, and essential oils. As with any herbal remedy, it is important to consult with a healthcare provider before using chamomile to treat any health condition.

Medicinal Chamomile Recipes

Here are a few medicinal chamomile recipes you can try:

Chamomile Tea: Chamomile tea is a popular and easy way to consume chamomile. To make the tea, steep 1-2 teaspoons of dried chamomile flowers in boiling water for 5-10 minutes, then strain and enjoy. You can add honey or lemon for added flavor.

Chamomile Salve: Chamomile salve can be used topically to soothe skin irritation, inflammation, and minor wounds. To make the salve, combine 1 cup of chamomile-infused oil (made by steeping chamomile flowers in oil for several weeks) with 1/4 cup of grated beeswax. Melt the beeswax in a double boiler, then add the chamomile oil and stir until well combined. Pour the mixture into small jars or tins and let cool.

Chamomile Bath: A chamomile bath can be a relaxing and soothing way to unwind after a long day. To make the bath, add 1 cup of dried chamomile flowers to a muslin bag or cheesecloth, and tie it closed. Fill the bathtub with warm water and add the chamomile bag, letting it steep for 10-15 minutes before soaking in the tub.

Simple Chamomile Tincture: Chamomile tincture is a concentrated form of chamomile that can be used to treat a variety of ailments. To make the tincture, fill a glass jar with dried chamomile flowers, then cover with vodka or another high-proof alcohol. Let the mixture steep for 4-6 weeks, shaking the jar occasionally. Strain the mixture through a cheesecloth or coffee filter, and store in a dark glass bottle.

Tincture at times can be hard to make so here is a more in depth recipe:

Ingredients:

- Dried chamomile flowers
- High-proof alcohol (such as vodka or grain alcohol)
- Glass jar with a tight-fitting lid
- Cheesecloth or fine-mesh sieve
- Amber glass dropper bottles for storage

Instructions:

1. Ensure your glass jar is clean and sterilized.

2. Fill the jar about one-third to one-half full with dried chamomile flowers.

3. Pour enough high-proof alcohol into the jar to completely cover the chamomile flowers. The alcohol should have a strength of at least 40% (80 proof) to effectively extract the plant's constituents.

4. Use a clean spoon or chopstick to stir the mixture, ensuring all the chamomile flowers are submerged in the alcohol.

5. Close the jar tightly with the lid.

6. Place the jar in a cool, dark place, such as a cupboard or pantry, and let it sit for 4 to 6 weeks. This allows for the maceration process, during which the alcohol extracts the beneficial compounds from the chamomile flowers. Shake the jar gently every few days to agitate the mixture.

7. After the maceration period, strain the liquid by pouring it through a cheesecloth or fine-mesh sieve into a clean bowl or another jar.

8. Squeeze the cheesecloth or press the plant material in the sieve to extract as much liquid as possible.

9. Pour the strained tincture into amber glass dropper bottles for storage. The amber glass helps protect the tincture from light, which can degrade its potency.

10. Label the bottles with the date and contents.

11. Store the chamomile tincture in a cool, dark place. It should remain potent for several years if stored properly.

To use the chamomile tincture, it can be taken orally by adding a few drops (usually 30-40 drops) to a glass of water or tea. It can also be used topically by diluting a few drops in a carrier oil and applying it to the skin. Chamomile tincture is known for its calming and soothing properties, often used to promote relaxation, support digestion, and alleviate minor skin irritations. Remember to consult with a healthcare professional or herbalist for appropriate dosage and usage instructions.

Cleavers (Galium aparine)

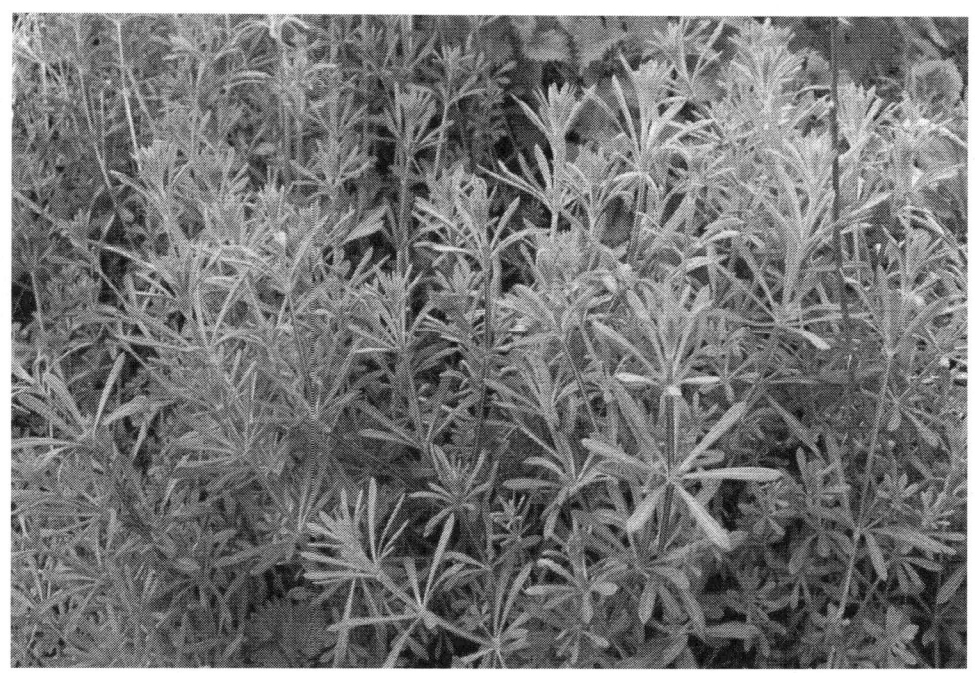

History of Galium Aparine

Galium aparine, commonly known as cleavers or sticky weed, has a long history of use in traditional medicine. The plant is native to Europe, North America, and parts of Asia, and has been used for centuries for its medicinal properties.

In traditional European medicine, cleavers were used as a diuretic to help eliminate excess fluids from the body and to treat skin conditions such as eczema and psoriasis. They were also used to support the lymphatic system and to help with conditions such as swollen lymph nodes and tonsillitis.

In North America, indigenous tribes used cleavers to treat urinary tract infections, as well as to relieve pain and inflammation associated with arthritis and other conditions.

Cleavers have also been used in traditional Chinese medicine, where they are known as "Qian Jin Zi," and are used to treat skin conditions, fevers, and as a diuretic.

Today, cleavers are still used in traditional medicine around the world and are often used as a natural remedy for conditions such as edema, skin irritations, and digestive issues. They are also commonly used in herbal teas and supplements, and can be found in health food stores and online retailers.

How to Grow Cleaver Plant

Cleavers, also known as Galium aparine, is a fast-growing, annual plant that is native to Europe and parts of Asia. Here are the steps to grow cleaver plant:

Choose a location: Cleavers grow well in partial shade to full sun and prefer a well-draining soil. They can tolerate a variety of soil types but grow best in fertile, moist soil.

Sow the seeds: Sow the cleaver seeds directly in the garden bed after the last frost date, about 1/4 inch deep and 2 inches apart. You can also start the seeds indoors 4-6 weeks before the last frost date and transplant them outside when they are about 3 inches tall.

Water the seeds: Water the seeds immediately after planting and keep the soil moist until the seedlings emerge. Once the seedlings have emerged, water them deeply once a week.

Thin the seedlings: When the seedlings are about 2-3 inches tall, thin them to one plant every 6-8 inches. This will give each plant enough space to grow and produce a good crop.

Fertilize: Cleavers do not require much fertilizer, but they can benefit from a light application of compost or well-rotted manure in the spring.

Harvest: Cleavers can be harvested once the plant has grown to about 6-8 inches tall. You can harvest the young leaves and stems, which are tender and have a slightly sweet taste. The plant also produces small, white flowers in the summer, which can be harvested and dried for use in herbal teas.

Overwinter: Cleavers are an annual plant, so they will die off after one growing season. However, they self-seed easily and may come back the following year on their own.

Cleavers can be a great addition to your garden, as they are easy to grow and have many medicinal properties. They are known for their ability to support the lymphatic system, and can be used as a diuretic and for skin conditions.

How to Clone Galium Aparine Plant

Galium aparine, or cleavers, can be propagated by taking stem cuttings. Here are the steps to clone a cleavers plant:

Choose a healthy and mature cleavers plant to take cuttings from. Look for a plant that has several stems and is at least 6 inches tall.

Cut several 4-6 inch stem cuttings from the cleavers plant. Make the cut just below a leaf node, which is the area where the leaves meet the stem. Strip off the lower leaves from the stem cuttings, leaving only the top few leaves.

Dip the cut end of each stem cutting into rooting hormone, which can be purchased from a garden center or online retailer. This will help to promote root growth.

Plant the stem cuttings in a pot or container filled with moist potting soil. Make a small hole in the soil with a pencil or your finger and insert the stem cutting, then gently firm the soil around the stem.

Water the soil to keep it moist, but not soaking wet. Keep the pot in a warm and humid location, such as a greenhouse or covered porch.

After a few weeks, the stem cuttings should start to develop roots. You can check for roots by gently tugging on the stem cutting. If you feel resistance, it means that roots have formed.

Once the stem cuttings have developed roots, you can transplant them into individual pots or into a garden bed. Be sure to water the new plants regularly and provide them with plenty of sunlight and nutrients.

With proper care and attention, your cleavers stem cuttings should grow into healthy and vigorous plants.

How is Galium Aparine Medicinal

Galium aparine, commonly known as cleavers, has a long history of medicinal use. Here are some of the medicinal properties and benefits associated with this plant:

Lymphatic support: Cleavers are known to support the lymphatic system, which is responsible for removing waste and toxins from the body. They are often used in traditional medicine to help with conditions such as swollen lymph nodes and tonsillitis.

Diuretic: Cleavers have a diuretic effect, which means that they can help to increase urine production and promote the elimination of excess fluids from the body. This can be helpful in cases of water retention and edema.

Skin conditions: Cleavers have been traditionally used to treat various skin conditions, such as psoriasis, eczema, and acne. They are believed to have anti-inflammatory and cleansing properties that can help to soothe and heal the skin.

Digestive support: Cleavers can be used to support digestion and relieve gastrointestinal issues, such as bloating, constipation, and indigestion. Anti-inflammatory: Cleavers contain compounds that have anti-inflammatory properties, which can help to reduce inflammation in the body and alleviate symptoms of inflammatory conditions, such as arthritis. Cleavers can be consumed as a tea, tincture, or in capsule form to reap the benefits of its medicinal properties. However, it is important to consult with a healthcare professional before using cleavers as a natural remedy, particularly if you are pregnant, breastfeeding, or taking medication.

Medicinal Cleaver Recipes

Cleavers, or Galium aparine, have a variety of medicinal uses, including as a diuretic, lymphatic system support, and skin healing. Here are a few recipes that use cleavers for their medicinal properties:

Cleavers Tea: To make cleavers tea, add 1-2 teaspoons of dried cleavers to a cup of boiling water. Allow the tea to steep for 10-15 minutes, then strain and drink. This tea can be consumed daily to support the lymphatic system and promote the elimination of excess fluids from the body.

Cleavers Poultice: To make a cleavers poultice, crush fresh cleavers leaves and stems in a mortar and pestle, then apply the paste directly to the affected area. Cover the poultice with a cloth or bandage to hold it in place, and leave it on for 20-30 minutes. This can be used to soothe skin irritations, rashes, and insect bites.

Cleavers Infused Oil: To make a cleavers infused oil, fill a glass jar with fresh or dried cleavers, then cover the plant material with a carrier oil such as olive oil or coconut oil. Seal the jar and allow it to sit in a sunny location for 4-6 weeks, shaking it occasionally. Strain the oil and store it in a dark bottle. This infused oil can be applied topically to soothe skin irritations and promote healing.

Cleavers Tincture: To make a cleavers tincture, fill a glass jar with fresh or dried cleavers, then cover the plant material with a high-proof alcohol such as vodka or brandy. Seal the jar and allow it to sit in a cool, dark location for 4-6 weeks, shaking it occasionally. Strain the tincture and store it in a dark bottle. This tincture can be taken internally to support the lymphatic system and promote the elimination of excess fluids from the body.

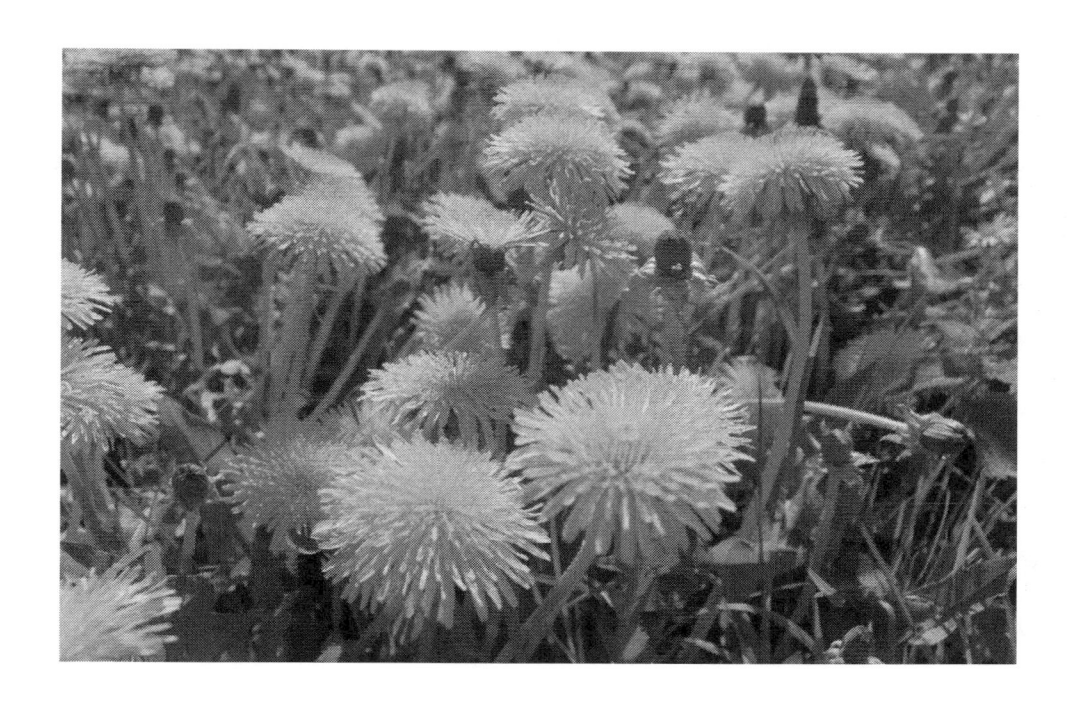

Dandelion

History of Dandelion

Dandelions have a long and fascinating history. Here are some key points: Origins: Dandelions are believed to have originated in Eurasia and have been cultivated for their medicinal and culinary properties for thousands of years.

Ancient Uses: The ancient Greeks and Romans used dandelions as a medicine to treat various ailments, including digestive issues, skin problems, and even depression. Dandelions were also commonly used in traditional Chinese medicine.

Medieval Europe: In the Middle Ages, dandelions were used to treat a variety of illnesses, including fever, boils, and eye problems. Dandelion wine was also a popular remedy for liver ailments.

Native American Uses: Native Americans used dandelions as a food source and medicine. The leaves were eaten as a salad green, and the roots were roasted and used as a coffee substitute.

Modern Uses: Dandelions are still widely used in herbal medicine today, and many people consider them a nutritious food source. Dandelion leaves and roots are said to have anti-inflammatory properties, and dandelion tea is often consumed to aid in digestion.

Symbolism: Dandelions have also been used as symbols of various things throughout history. In medieval times, they were considered a symbol of faithfulness and loyalty. Today, they are often seen as a symbol of hope and resilience, as they can thrive in even the most challenging environments.

Overall, dandelions have a rich and varied history and continue to be an important plant in many cultures and traditions.

How to Grow Dandelion

Dandelions are easy to grow and will thrive in most soil types and climates.

Here are the steps to grow dandelion:

Choose a planting location: Dandelions prefer full sun but can also grow in partial shade. They will grow in almost any type of soil but prefer well-draining soil that is rich in nutrients.

Plant dandelion seeds: Dandelion seeds can be purchased from a garden center or online. Scatter the seeds over the planting area and lightly cover them with soil. Water the seeds thoroughly after planting.

Water regularly: Keep the soil consistently moist but not waterlogged. Dandelions are drought-tolerant but will produce more leaves if they are well-watered.

Fertilize occasionally: Dandelions are heavy feeders and will benefit from a nitrogen-rich fertilizer. Apply fertilizer once a month during the growing season.

Harvest the leaves: Dandelion leaves can be harvested when they are young and tender, usually in the spring and fall. Use a sharp knife or scissors to cut the leaves off at the base of the plant.

Control the spread: Dandelions are a fast-spreading plant and can quickly take over a garden if left unchecked. To prevent them from spreading, remove any yellow flowers before they turn into fluffy seed heads.

Note: If you want to prevent dandelions from spreading in your lawn, you can mow them regularly or use an herbicide specifically designed to kill dandelions.

How to Clone Dandelion Plants

Cloning dandelion plants is relatively easy, and there are two main methods to do so:

Root Cuttings: This method involves taking a cutting of the dandelion root and planting it in soil. Here are the steps:

Choose a healthy dandelion plant with a well-developed root system. Using a sharp knife or scissors, cut a section of the root from the parent plant. The cutting should be about 2-3 inches long.

Plant the cutting in a container filled with potting soil, burying it about 1 inch deep.

Water the cutting gently to moisten the soil and place it in a warm, sunny location.

Keep the soil moist and wait for the cutting to develop new growth.

Leaf Cuttings: This method involves taking a cutting of the dandelion leaves and planting them in soil. Here are the steps:

Choose a healthy dandelion plant with a well-developed leaf system. Using a sharp knife or scissors, cut a section of the leaves from the parent plant. The cutting should include a small section of the stem.

Plant the cutting in a container filled with potting soil, burying it about 1/4 inch deep.

Water the cutting gently to moisten the soil and place it in a warm, sunny location.

Keep the soil moist and wait for the cutting to develop new growth.

In both methods, it's important to keep the soil moist and the cutting in a warm, sunny location. Once the cutting has developed new growth, it can be transplanted to a larger pot or planted directly in the ground.

How is Dandelion Medicinal

Dandelions have been used for their medicinal properties for centuries. Here are some of the ways in which dandelions are believed to be beneficial for health:

Digestive Health: Dandelions are believed to stimulate the production of digestive juices, which can help to improve digestion and relieve constipation. Dandelion tea is often used as a natural remedy for upset stomach, heartburn, and bloating.

Liver Health: Dandelion root has been traditionally used to support liver function and treat liver diseases. Dandelion is believed to stimulate the liver and gallbladder, which can help to improve bile production and digestion. Anti-Inflammatory: Dandelion contains compounds called sesquiterpene lactones, which have been shown to have anti-inflammatory effects. This makes dandelion useful in treating conditions such as arthritis and other inflammatory disorders.

Diuretic: Dandelion has diuretic properties, which means it can help to increase urine production and remove excess water from the body. This makes dandelion useful in treating conditions such as high blood pressure, edema, and urinary tract infections.

Antioxidant: Dandelion contains antioxidants, which can help to protect the body against damage from free radicals. This makes dandelion useful in preventing chronic diseases such as cancer, heart disease, and diabetes. Skin Health: Dandelion has been used topically to treat skin conditions such as acne, eczema, and psoriasis. Dandelion is believed to have anti-inflammatory and antibacterial properties, which can help to soothe and heal irritated skin.

It's important to note that while dandelions have been used for medicinal purposes for centuries, more research is needed to fully understand their potential health benefits and any potential risks or side effects. As with any natural remedy, it's always a good idea to talk to your healthcare provider before using dandelion or any other herbal supplement.

Medicinal Recipes with Dandelion

Dandelion is a versatile plant that can be used in a variety of medicinal recipes. Here are a few examples:

Dandelion Tea: Dandelion tea is easy to make and is a popular natural remedy for digestive issues. Here's how to make it: Boil 1 cup of water in a small pot or kettle.

Add 1 teaspoon of dried dandelion leaves or 2 teaspoons of fresh dandelion leaves to a tea infuser or tea ball.

Place the tea infuser or tea ball in a mug and pour the boiling water over it.

Let the tea steep for 5-10 minutes, then remove the tea infuser or tea ball.

If desired, add honey or lemon to taste.

Dandelion Salve: Dandelion salve is a topical ointment that can be used to soothe and heal irritated skin. Here's how to make it:

Combine 1 cup of dandelion flowers with 1 cup of olive oil in a small pot or slow cooker.

Heat the mixture on low for several hours, stirring occasionally, until the oil is infused with the dandelion flowers.

Strain the oil through a cheesecloth or fine mesh sieve, discarding the flowers.

Return the infused oil to the pot or slow cooker and add 1/4 cup of beeswax.

Heat the mixture on low, stirring occasionally, until the beeswax is melted and the mixture is smooth.

Pour the mixture into a clean jar or tin and let it cool and solidify. Dandelion Tincture: Dandelion tincture is a concentrated liquid extract that can be used to treat a variety of health conditions. Here's how to make it: Fill a jar with chopped dandelion roots or leaves (or a combination of both). Cover the plant material with high-proof alcohol (such as vodka or brandy). Cap the jar tightly and shake it well.

Store the jar in a cool, dark place for 4-6 weeks, shaking it occasionally. Strain the liquid through a cheesecloth or fine mesh sieve, discarding the plant material.

Pour the tincture into a clean bottle or jar and store it in a cool, dark place. As with any herbal remedy, it's important to consult with a healthcare provider before using dandelion or any other plant for medicinal purposes.

Dandelion recipe

Dandelion salad recipe

Here's a simple recipe for a delicious dandelion salad:

Ingredients:

- 1 bunch of fresh dandelion greens
- 1 small red onion, sliced
- 1/2 cup of crumbled feta cheese
- 1/4 cup of chopped walnuts
- 2 tablespoons of extra-virgin olive oil
- 1 tablespoon of apple cider vinegar
- 1 teaspoon of Dijon mustard
- Salt and pepper to taste

Instructions:

Wash and dry the dandelion greens and chop them into bite-sized pieces. In a small bowl, whisk together the olive oil, apple cider vinegar, Dijon mustard, salt, and pepper to make the dressing.

In a large mixing bowl, combine the chopped dandelion greens, sliced red onion, crumbled feta cheese, and chopped walnuts.

Pour the dressing over the salad and toss everything together until the greens are evenly coated.

Serve the salad immediately and enjoy!

Note: You can also add other ingredients to the salad, such as sliced apples or pears, cherry tomatoes, or grilled chicken, to make it more filling and flavorful.

Dong Quai
(Angelica sinensis)

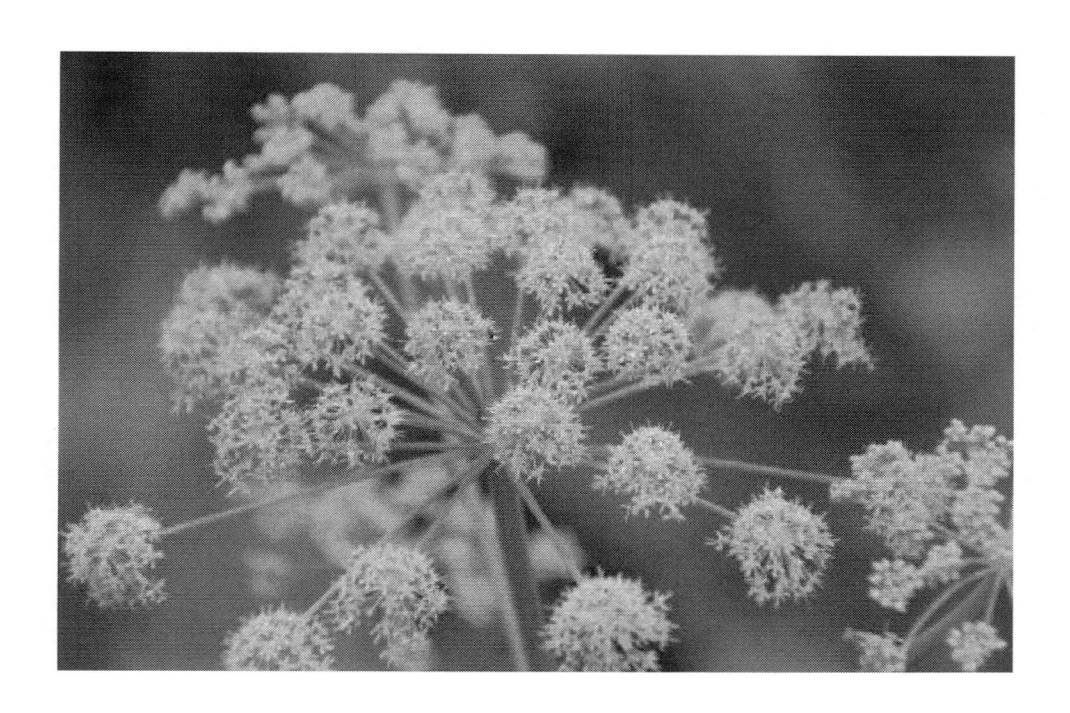

History of Dong Quai

Dong quai, also known as Angelica sinensis, is a traditional Chinese herb that has been used for over a thousand years to treat a variety of health conditions. The herb is believed to have originated in China and was first recorded in the ancient Chinese text, the Divine Farmer's Materia Medica, around 200 BCE.

In traditional Chinese medicine, dong quai is considered a blood tonic and is commonly used to treat conditions related to the female reproductive system, such as menstrual cramps, irregular periods, and menopausal symptoms. It is also used to improve circulation, strengthen the immune system, and alleviate digestive problems.

Dong quai was introduced to Europe in the 17th century and quickly became popular as a medicinal herb. It was widely used in Europe during the 19th century to treat various conditions such as anemia, headache, and rheumatism.

In modern times, dong quai has gained popularity as a natural remedy for menopausal symptoms, particularly hot flashes and vaginal dryness. It is also used as an ingredient in some skincare products due to its purported ability to improve skin health.

While dong quai has a long history of use in traditional Chinese medicine and is generally considered safe, it may interact with certain medications and should be used with caution in some individuals. As with any herbal supplement, it is important to consult with a healthcare professional before use.

How to Grow Dong Quai

Dong quai (Angelica sinensis) is a hardy perennial herb that can be grown in USDA plant hardiness zones 4-9. Here are the steps to grow dong quai:

Soil: Dong quai grows best in well-draining soil that is rich in organic matter. Amend the soil with compost or well-rotted manure before planting to improve soil fertility and texture.

Sunlight: Dong quai prefers partial shade to full shade. It can tolerate some direct sunlight in cooler climates, but too much sun can cause the leaves to wilt and dry out.

Watering: Dong quai requires regular watering to keep the soil moist but not waterlogged. Water deeply once or twice a week during dry periods to prevent the soil from drying out.

Fertilizer: Fertilize dong quai with a balanced fertilizer once or twice a year, preferably in early spring and late summer.

Propagation: Dong quai can be propagated by seed or stem cuttings. Seeds should be sown in early spring, while stem cuttings can be taken in late summer.

Maintenance: Dong quai is a slow-growing plant that requires minimal maintenance. Remove any dead or yellowing leaves to prevent the spread of diseases.

Harvesting: Dong quai is usually harvested in the fall when the roots are fully developed. To harvest, dig up the entire plant and carefully remove the roots. Wash the roots thoroughly and allow them to dry in a warm, well-ventilated area for several days.

It is important to note that dong quai may interact with certain medications and should be used with caution in some individuals. Always consult with a healthcare professional before using dong quai for medicinal purposes.

How to Clone Dong Quai

Dong quai (Angelica sinensis) can be propagated through seed or stem cuttings. Here is how to clone dong quai using stem cuttings:

Select a healthy dong quai plant that is at least one year old. Choose a stem that is at least 6 inches long and has several leaves.

Cut the stem with a sharp, sterile knife just below a node (a point where leaves grow out of the stem).

Remove the leaves from the lower half of the stem, leaving a few leaves at the top.

Dip the cut end of the stem in rooting hormone powder to encourage root growth.

Plant the stem cutting in a pot filled with moist potting soil. Make a small hole in the soil with a pencil and insert the stem cutting.

Cover the pot with a plastic bag to create a humid environment and place it in a warm, bright location.

Check the soil moisture regularly and water as needed to keep the soil moist but not waterlogged.

After a few weeks, the cutting should start to develop roots. Once the roots are established, the plant can be transplanted into a larger pot or planted outdoors in a sunny, well-drained location.

It is important to note that dong quai is a slow-growing plant and can take several years to mature. It requires rich, well-drained soil and regular watering. Additionally, as with any herbal supplement, it is recommended to consult with a healthcare professional before using dong quai for medicinal purposes.

How is Dong Quai Medicinal

Dong quai (Angelica sinensis) has been traditionally used as a medicinal herb in Chinese medicine for thousands of years. It is considered to have a range of health benefits, including:

Regulating menstrual cycle: Dong quai has been used to regulate the menstrual cycle and alleviate menstrual pain and cramps. It contains compounds that can help relax the uterus and promote blood flow, which can help ease these symptoms.

Reducing menopausal symptoms: Dong quai is often used to alleviate hot flashes, vaginal dryness, and other symptoms associated with menopause. It contains phytoestrogens, which are plant-based compounds that can mimic the effects of estrogen in the body and help balance hormone levels. Improving circulation: Dong quai is believed to improve blood circulation and oxygen delivery throughout the body. It can help improve energy levels, reduce fatigue, and promote overall vitality.

Boosting immune system: Dong quai is believed to have immune-boosting properties. It contains compounds that can help stimulate the production of white blood cells and enhance the body's ability to fight off infections and diseases.

Alleviating pain: Dong quai has been traditionally used to alleviate various types of pain, including headaches, joint pain, and muscle pain. It contains anti-inflammatory compounds that can help reduce inflammation and relieve pain.

Dong quai is available in various forms, including teas, capsules, and tinctures. However, it is important to note that dong quai may interact with certain medications and should be used with caution in some individuals. It is always recommended to consult with a healthcare professional before using any herbal supplement.

Medicinal Recipes for Dong Quai

Dong quai (Angelica sinensis) is a traditional Chinese herb that has been used for medicinal purposes for thousands of years. Here are a few medicinal recipes that include dong quai:

Dong Quai Tea for Menstrual Cramps:

- 1 tablespoon dried dong quai root
- 1 tablespoon dried ginger root
- 1 tablespoon dried chamomile flowers
- 3 cups water

Instructions:

Boil the water in a pot and add the dried herbs.

Reduce the heat and simmer for 15-20 minutes.

Strain the tea and drink 1-2 cups per day during menstruation to alleviate menstrual cramps.

Dong Quai and Goji Berry Tonic for Immune System:

- 1 tablespoon dried dong quai root
- 1 tablespoon dried goji berries
- 2 cups water
- Honey (optional)

Instructions:

Boil the water in a pot and add the dried herbs.

Reduce the heat and simmer for 20-30 minutes.

Strain the tonic and add honey to taste (if desired).

Drink 1-2 cups per day to boost the immune system.

Dong Quai and Red Date Soup for Blood Tonic:

- 6-8 dried red dates (jujubes)
- 1 tablespoon dried dong quai root
- 4 cups water
- Rock sugar (to taste)

Instructions:

Rinse the red dates and dong quai root.

Put them in a pot with 4 cups of water and bring to a boil.

Reduce the heat and simmer for 30-40 minutes.

Add rock sugar to taste (if desired).

Drink 1-2 cups per day to tonify the blood.

Note: These recipes are for informational purposes only and should not be used as a substitute for professional medical advice. Always consult with a healthcare provider before using any herbal remedies.

Echinacea

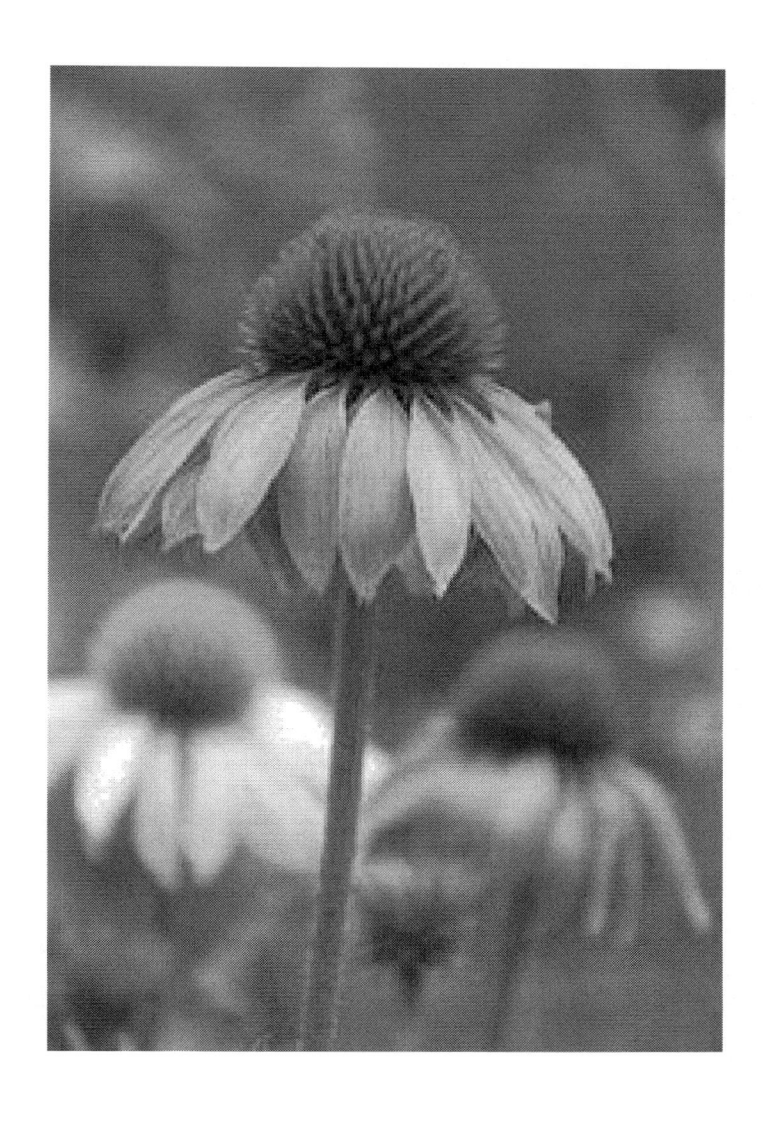

History of Echinacea

Echinacea, also known as the purple coneflower, is a group of flowering plants in the daisy family native to North America. The plant has a long history of use among Native American tribes for its medicinal properties.

The use of Echinacea as a medicinal herb can be traced back to the 18th and 19th centuries when European settlers learned about the plant from the Native Americans. The Plains Indians used Echinacea to treat a variety of ailments, including toothaches, sore throats, coughs, and wounds. They also used it as a general tonic to boost the immune system.

Echinacea was first introduced to Europe in the late 1800s, where it gained popularity as a natural remedy. In the early 1900s, it was included in the official pharmacopeias of several European countries.

In the United States, Echinacea became widely used as a natural remedy during the 20th century. The popularity of Echinacea surged in the 1990s, with sales of Echinacea supplements reaching millions of dollars.

Today, Echinacea is one of the most popular herbal supplements in the world and is used to support the immune system, reduce inflammation, and treat a variety of conditions, including the common cold, flu, and respiratory infections.

How to Grow Echinacea

Echinacea, also known as coneflower, is a perennial herb that is easy to grow in most regions. Here are some steps to grow Echinacea:

Choose a location: Echinacea grows best in full sun to partial shade, and prefers well-drained soil. Choose a location that gets at least 6 hours of sunlight per day and has soil that drains well.

Prepare the soil: Before planting, amend the soil with compost or well-rotted manure to improve drainage and add nutrients. Echinacea prefers soil with a pH between 6.0 and 7.0.

Plant the seeds or seedlings: Echinacea can be started from seed indoors in late winter or early spring, or sown directly in the ground in early spring. Plant seeds ¼ inch deep and water lightly. Seedlings can also be planted in the ground after the last frost.

Water regularly: Echinacea prefers evenly moist soil, so water regularly and deeply, especially during hot and dry weather.

Mulch: Mulch around the plants with a layer of organic material, such as shredded leaves or straw, to help retain moisture in the soil and keep weeds under control.

Deadhead regularly: To encourage continuous blooming, deadhead spent flowers regularly by cutting the stem back to a leaf node. This will also help prevent the plant from self-seeding too much.

Divide the plants: Echinacea can become crowded after a few years and may need to be divided to maintain healthy growth. Dig up the plants in the fall, separate the clumps, and replant in a new location or give away to friends.

By following these steps, you should be able to grow Echinacea successfully and enjoy its beautiful blooms and medicinal benefits.

How to Clone Echinacea

Echinacea can be propagated through stem cuttings or division. To propagate Echinacea through stem cuttings, follow these steps: Choose a healthy plant: Choose a healthy Echinacea plant with strong stems and healthy leaves.

Cut a stem: Cut a stem from the plant that is about 4 to 6 inches long, with a sharp, clean pair of scissors or pruning shears.

Remove leaves: Remove the lower leaves from the stem, leaving only a few leaves near the top.

Dip in rooting hormone: Dip the cut end of the stem in rooting hormone powder or gel, which will help promote root growth.

Plant the cutting: Plant the cutting in a container filled with moist soilless potting mix or a mix of sand and peat moss.

Cover with plastic: Cover the container with a plastic bag or a plastic dome to create a humid environment.

Water and care: Water the cutting regularly, keeping the soil moist but not waterlogged. Place the container in a warm, bright location, but out of direct sunlight.

Wait for roots to form: After several weeks, check for root development by gently tugging on the stem. If you feel resistance, roots have formed and the plant is ready to be transplanted into a larger container or the garden. To propagate Echinacea through division, follow these steps:

Dig up the plant: In the fall, dig up the entire Echinacea plant, being careful not to damage the roots.

Separate the clumps: Use a sharp, clean pair of scissors or a garden knife to separate the clumps of roots into smaller sections. Each section should have at least one healthy root system and several stems.

Replant: Replant the divisions in a new location, spacing them at least 12 inches apart. Water them thoroughly and add a layer of mulch around the plants to help retain moisture in the soil.

By following these steps, you can successfully clone or propagate Echinacea and expand your garden or share with friends.

How is Echinacea Medicinal

Echinacea is a popular herbal remedy that is believed to have many health benefits. It is commonly used to support the immune system and to help prevent and treat the common cold, flu, and other respiratory infections. Here are some of the ways that Echinacea is believed to be medicinal:

Boosts the immune system: Echinacea is believed to stimulate the immune system, which can help the body fight off infections and other illnesses. Reduces inflammation: Echinacea has anti-inflammatory properties, which can help reduce inflammation in the body and relieve pain.

Helps prevent and treat the common cold: Echinacea is often used to prevent and treat the common cold. It may help reduce the severity and duration of cold symptoms.

May help treat respiratory infections: Echinacea is believed to have antiviral and antibacterial properties, which may make it helpful in treating respiratory infections, such as bronchitis and sinusitis.

May help with skin conditions: Echinacea is believed to have anti-inflammatory and antimicrobial properties, which may make it helpful in treating skin conditions such as eczema and psoriasis.

May help with anxiety and depression: Some studies suggest that Echinacea may have a mild calming effect and may be helpful in reducing anxiety and depression.

Echinacea is available in many forms, including capsules, teas, tinctures, and creams. It is important to talk to your healthcare provider before taking Echinacea, especially if you have any medical conditions or are taking other medications.

Medicinal Echinacea Recipes

Here are some medicinal recipes using Echinacea:

Echinacea Tea: Add 1-2 teaspoons of dried Echinacea leaves or flowers to a cup of boiling water. Steep for 10-15 minutes, strain, and drink. You can add honey or lemon to taste.

Echinacea Tincture: Combine 1 part dried Echinacea root or leaves with 2 parts 100 proof vodka in a glass jar. Shake daily for 4-6 weeks, then strain and store in a dark glass dropper bottle. Take 30-40 drops in water, 3 times a day when needed.

Echinacea Salve: Melt 1/4 cup of beeswax and 1/2 cup of coconut oil in a double boiler. Add 1/2 cup of dried Echinacea flowers and leaves, and let simmer for 20-30 minutes. Strain and pour into jars. Apply to minor cuts and scrapes as needed.

Echinacea and Honey Cough Syrup: Combine 1/2 cup of honey with 1/2 cup of warm water in a glass jar. Add 1 tablespoon of dried Echinacea leaves or flowers, and let steep for 4-6 hours. Strain and store in a jar. Take 1 teaspoon as needed for coughs and sore throat.

It's important to note that Echinacea is not recommended for everyone. It can interact with certain medications, and it may not be safe for people with certain medical conditions, such as autoimmune diseases or allergies to plants in the daisy family.

Feverfew

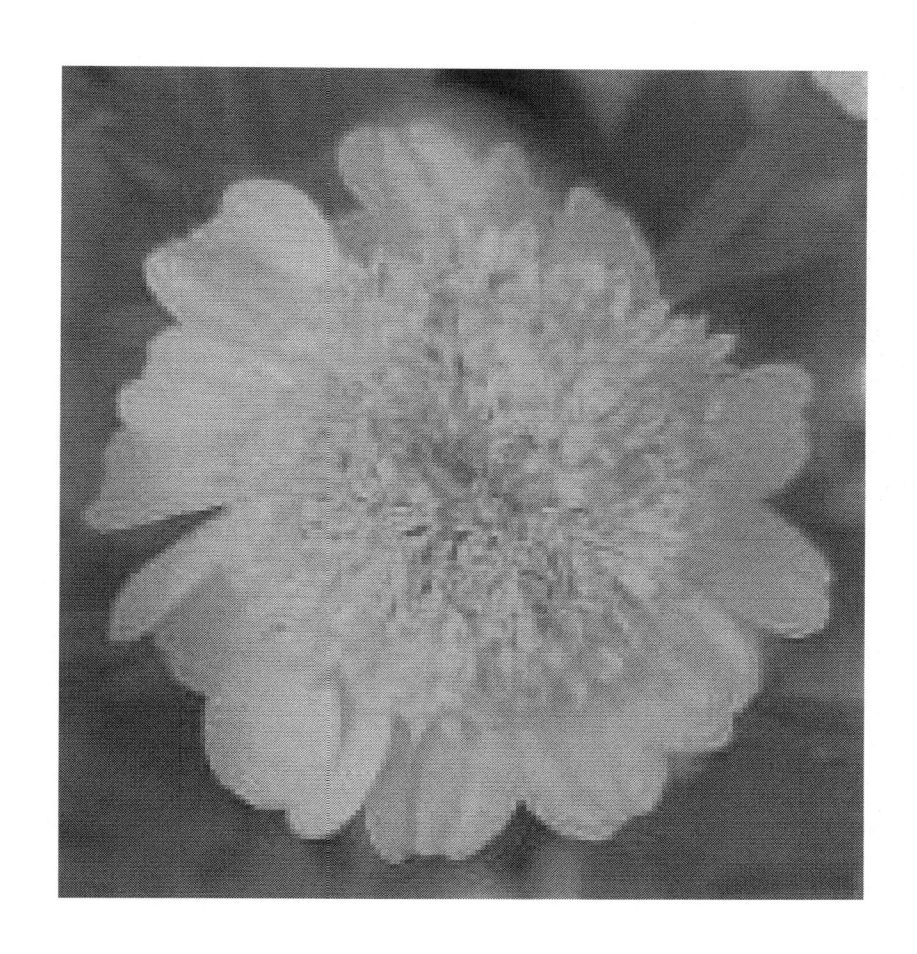

History of Feverfew Plant

Feverfew, also known as featherfew or bachelor's button, is a herbaceous plant belonging to the daisy family, Asteraceae. It is native to southeastern Europe but is now widely cultivated in other parts of the world, including North America. The plant has a long history of use in traditional medicine, dating back to ancient Greece, where it was used to treat a variety of ailments, including fever, headaches, and arthritis. It was also used in medieval times to treat menstrual disorders and relieve labor pains. In the 1970s, feverfew gained popularity as a treatment for migraines, and its use for this purpose has continued to the present day

How to Grow Feverfew

Feverfew is a plant that belongs to the daisy family and is commonly grown for its medicinal properties. Here are some tips on how to grow feverfew:

Choose a location: Feverfew grows best in full sun to partial shade. It prefers well-draining soil that is rich in organic matter.

Start from seed: You can start feverfew from seed indoors about 6-8 weeks before the last frost date. Sow the seeds in a well-draining soil mix and cover them lightly with soil. Keep the soil moist and warm until the seeds germinate.

Transplant outdoors: Once the seedlings have grown a few sets of leaves, you can transplant them outdoors. Choose a spot that receives full sun to partial shade, and has well-draining soil. Space the plants about 12-18 inches apart.

Water regularly: Feverfew needs regular watering, especially during the hot summer months. Water the plants deeply once a week or more often if the soil is dry.

Fertilize: You can fertilize feverfew with a balanced, all-purpose fertilizer once or twice a month during the growing season.

Harvest the leaves: You can harvest the leaves of feverfew as needed once the plant has grown to a decent size. The leaves can be used fresh or dried for medicinal purposes.

Propagate through division: Feverfew can be propagated through division in the fall or early spring. Dig up the plant and gently separate the roots into smaller sections. Replant the smaller sections in well-draining soil and water regularly until they establish themselves.

With proper care, feverfew can grow up to 2-3 feet tall and produce beautiful daisy-like flowers in the summer.

How to Clone Feverfew Plant

Feverfew can be propagated through stem cuttings, division, and seeds.

Here's how to clone feverfew plant using stem cuttings:

Choose a healthy feverfew plant with no signs of disease or insect damage. Take stem cuttings in early spring or summer, using sharp and clean gardening shears.

Cut a stem about 4-6 inches long with several sets of leaves.

Remove the lower sets of leaves, leaving only the top 2-3 sets of leaves intact.

Dip the cut end in rooting hormone powder to encourage root growth. Plant the stem cutting in a container filled with moist, well-draining soil or in a small hole in the garden.

Water the cutting regularly and keep it in a warm, bright location with partial shade for a few weeks until roots develop and new growth appears. Transplant the new feverfew plant into a larger pot or the garden once it has established itself. Propagation by division can also be done in the fall or early spring when the plant is dormant. Simply dig up the plant, separate the roots into several clumps, and plant each clump in a new location.

How is Feverfew Medicinal

Feverfew has been traditionally used for centuries for its medicinal properties. It is primarily used to treat headaches, especially migraines, and to reduce fever. Feverfew has also been used to treat arthritis, digestive disorders, and menstrual irregularities.

Feverfew contains a variety of biologically active compounds, including parthenolide, which has been shown to have anti-inflammatory and pain-relieving effects. It is believed to work by inhibiting the production of prostaglandins, which are hormone-like substances that contribute to inflammation and pain.

Feverfew is also believed to have antiplatelet and vasodilatory effects, which may help to reduce the frequency and severity of migraines. Additionally, it has been shown to have antioxidant properties, which may help to protect cells from damage caused by free radicals.

While feverfew is generally considered safe when used as directed, it may interact with certain medications and should not be used by pregnant or breastfeeding women without first consulting a healthcare provider.

Medicinal Feverfew Recipes

Feverfew is a herb with many medicinal properties, and it is used to treat a variety of health conditions. Here are some medicinal feverfew recipes:

Feverfew Tea: Boil a cup of water and add 1-2 teaspoons of dried feverfew leaves. Let it steep for 5-10 minutes, then strain the tea and add honey or lemon juice to taste.

Feverfew Tincture: Fill a jar with fresh feverfew leaves and pour alcohol over them until the jar is full. Let the jar sit in a cool, dark place for 4-6 weeks, shaking it occasionally. Strain the liquid into a clean jar and take 5-10 drops of the tincture up to three times a day.

Feverfew Capsules: Grind dried feverfew leaves into a fine powder and fill empty capsules with the powder. Take 1-2 capsules up to three times a day. Feverfew Salve: Melt 1/4 cup of beeswax in a double boiler, and add 1/2 cup of olive oil and 1/2 cup of dried feverfew leaves. Heat the mixture for 1-2 hours, then strain the liquid through cheesecloth into a clean jar. Add a few drops of essential oil if desired, then let the salve cool and solidify. Feverfew Compress: Steep a handful of fresh feverfew leaves in boiling water for 10-15 minutes, then strain the liquid and soak a clean cloth in it. Apply the damp cloth to the affected area and let it sit for 10-15 minutes. Repeat as needed.

Ginger

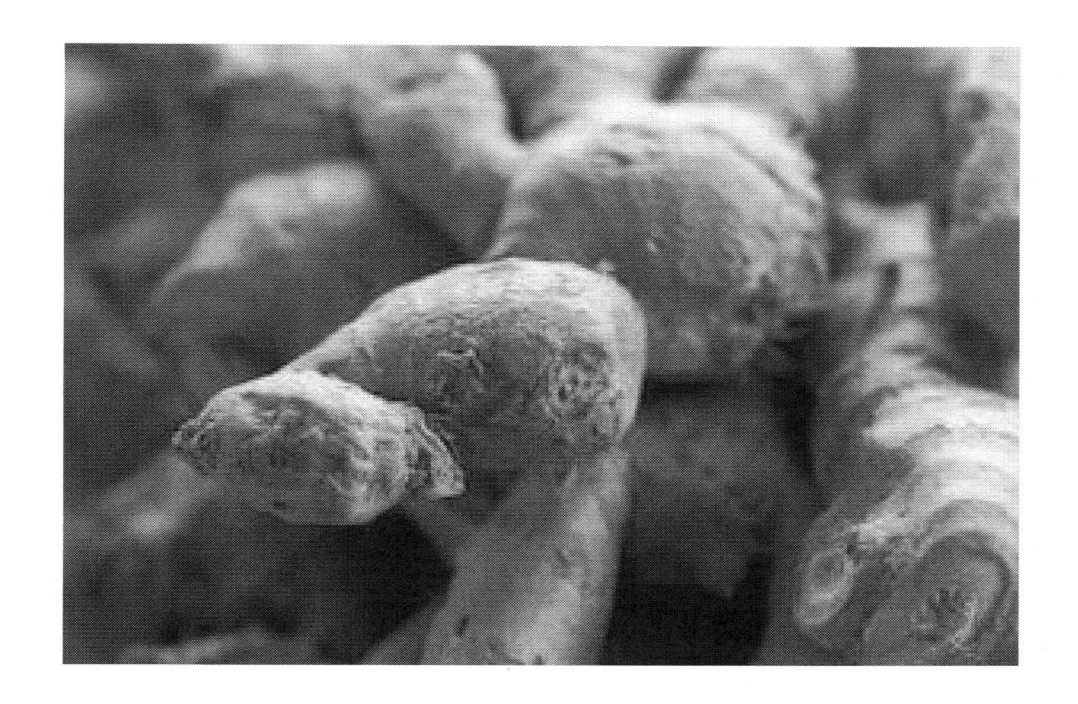

History of Ginger

Ginger (Zingiber officinale) has a long and rich history that dates back over 5,000 years. It is believed to have originated in Southeast Asia and was eventually traded throughout the ancient world. Here are some key historical facts about ginger:

Ancient China: Ginger was first cultivated in ancient China, where it was highly prized for its medicinal properties. It was also used as a spice to flavor food and as a key ingredient in traditional Chinese medicine. Ancient Rome: Ginger was introduced to Europe by the Romans, who used it as a spice and medicine.

Middle Ages: During the Middle Ages, ginger was a popular spice in Europe and was used to flavor food and drink. It was also used as a medicinal herb to treat a variety of ailments.

Renaissance: Ginger became more widely available in Europe during the Renaissance, and it was used to flavor sweets, such as gingerbread and ginger snaps.

18th and 19th centuries: Ginger became an important trade commodity during the 18th and 19th centuries. It was cultivated in tropical regions around the world, including the Caribbean and South America.

Today, ginger is used around the world for its culinary and medicinal properties. It is commonly used to treat digestive issues, such as nausea and indigestion, and is also used as a natural remedy for colds and flu.

How to Grow Ginger

Here are some steps to grow ginger:

Choose a ginger root: Look for a plump ginger root with tight skin and a few eye buds (similar to those on a potato). Avoid ginger roots that are shriveled, moldy, or have soft spots.

Soak the ginger: Soak the ginger root in water overnight to help it sprout.

Prepare a pot: Choose a pot that is at least 12 inches wide and 12 inches deep. Fill it with a well-draining potting mix that has been enriched with compost.

Plant the ginger: Plant the ginger root 2-4 inches deep, with the eye buds facing up. Cover with soil and water gently.

Water and care: Keep the soil consistently moist, but not waterlogged. Ginger likes warm and humid conditions, so consider placing the pot in a warm spot with bright, indirect light. You can also mist the plant with a spray bottle to increase humidity.

Harvesting: Ginger takes several months to mature. Once the plant is about 8-10 inches tall, you can start harvesting small pieces of ginger by gently pulling back the soil and cutting off a piece. Be sure to leave some of the roots intact so that the plant can continue to grow.

Repeat: Ginger is a perennial plant, so with proper care, it can produce a new crop every year. After harvesting, replant any remaining pieces of ginger and start the process again.

Growing ginger is a rewarding experience that can also be used for culinary and medicinal purposes.

Can You Clone Ginger?

Yes, it is possible to clone ginger. Here are the steps:

Choose a ginger rhizome: Select a fresh ginger rhizome that has several buds or eyes.

Cut the rhizome: Using a clean, sharp knife, cut the ginger rhizome into several sections, making sure each section has at least one bud or eye. Prepare a pot: Fill a pot with a well-draining potting mix that has been enriched with compost.

Plant the ginger: Plant each section of the ginger rhizome about 2 inches deep in the pot, with the bud or eye facing up. Cover with soil and water gently.

Water and care: Keep the soil consistently moist, but not waterlogged. Ginger likes warm and humid conditions, so consider placing the pot in a warm spot with bright, indirect light. You can also mist the plant with a spray bottle to increase humidity.

Wait for growth: Ginger can take several weeks to sprout. Be patient and keep the soil moist.

Transplant: Once the ginger has grown to about 6 inches tall, you can transplant it into a larger pot or outside into the ground.

By cloning ginger, you can create multiple plants from a single rhizome, making it an economical way to expand your ginger garden.

How is Ginger Medicinal?

Ginger has several medicinal properties and has been used for centuries to treat various ailments. Here are some of the ways ginger is used medicinally:

Anti-inflammatory: Ginger contains compounds called gingerols and shogaols, which have anti-inflammatory properties. These compounds can help reduce inflammation in the body, which can help relieve pain and swelling associated with conditions such as osteoarthritis, rheumatoid arthritis, and other inflammatory disorders.

Digestive aid: Ginger is commonly used to treat digestive issues such as nausea, vomiting, and indigestion. It can also help stimulate digestion, increase the production of digestive juices, and reduce intestinal gas. Immune system booster: Ginger has immune-boosting properties and can help strengthen the body's immune system. It can also help reduce the risk of infections by preventing the growth of harmful bacteria and viruses. Respiratory health: Ginger has anti-inflammatory and anti-viral properties that make it useful in treating respiratory illnesses such as colds and flu. It can help relieve congestion and reduce inflammation in the airways. Menstrual pain relief: Ginger can help relieve menstrual pain and cramps due to its anti-inflammatory properties.

Ginger can be consumed in many forms, including fresh ginger root, ginger tea, ginger supplements, and ginger oil. It is generally safe for most people when consumed in moderate amounts, but as with any supplement or medication, it is important to consult with a healthcare provider before using ginger medicinally.

Medicinal Ginger Recipe

Here's a simple medicinal ginger tea recipe that you can make at home:

Ingredients:

- 2-3 slices of fresh ginger root
- 1-2 cups of water
- 1-2 teaspoons of honey (optional)

Instructions:

Peel and slice the fresh ginger root into thin slices.

Bring water to a boil in a small pot.

Add the ginger slices to the boiling water.

Reduce the heat to low and let the ginger simmer for 10-15 minutes.

Remove the pot from heat and let it cool for a few minutes.

Strain the tea into a cup and add honey, if desired.

Enjoy your warm and soothing ginger tea!

This ginger tea can help relieve nausea, indigestion, and menstrual cramps. It is also a great immune booster, especially during cold and flu season. If you prefer a stronger flavor, you can add more ginger slices to the water. You can also add other herbs, such as lemon or mint, for added flavor and medicinal benefits.

Medicinal Ginger Recipes

Here are a few more medicinal ginger recipes:

Ginger and Turmeric Tea: Turmeric is also a powerful anti-inflammatory herb that works well with ginger. To make the tea, add 2-3 slices of fresh ginger and 1-2 teaspoons of turmeric powder to a cup of boiling water. Let it steep for 10-15 minutes, strain, and enjoy. You can also add honey and lemon for extra flavor.

Ginger and Garlic Soup: Garlic has antibacterial and antiviral properties that can help fight off infections. To make the soup, sauté 2-3 cloves of minced garlic and 2-3 slices of fresh ginger in a pot with a tablespoon of olive oil. Add 4 cups of chicken or vegetable broth and bring to a boil. Add chopped vegetables of your choice, such as carrots, celery, and kale, and let the soup simmer for 20-30 minutes. Season with salt and pepper to taste.

Ginger and Honey Syrup: This syrup can be used to soothe sore throats and coughs. To make it, grate 1-2 inches of fresh ginger and mix it with 1 cup of honey in a jar. Let it sit for a few hours to allow the ginger to infuse into the honey. Take 1-2 teaspoons of the syrup as needed.

Ginger and Lemon Shot: This is a quick and easy way to boost your immune system. Juice half a lemon and grate 1-2 inches of fresh ginger. Mix the juice and ginger in a shot glass and drink it straight up. You can also dilute it with water or add honey for taste.

Remember to always consult with a healthcare provider before using ginger medicinally, especially if you have any underlying health conditions or are taking medications.

Gingko

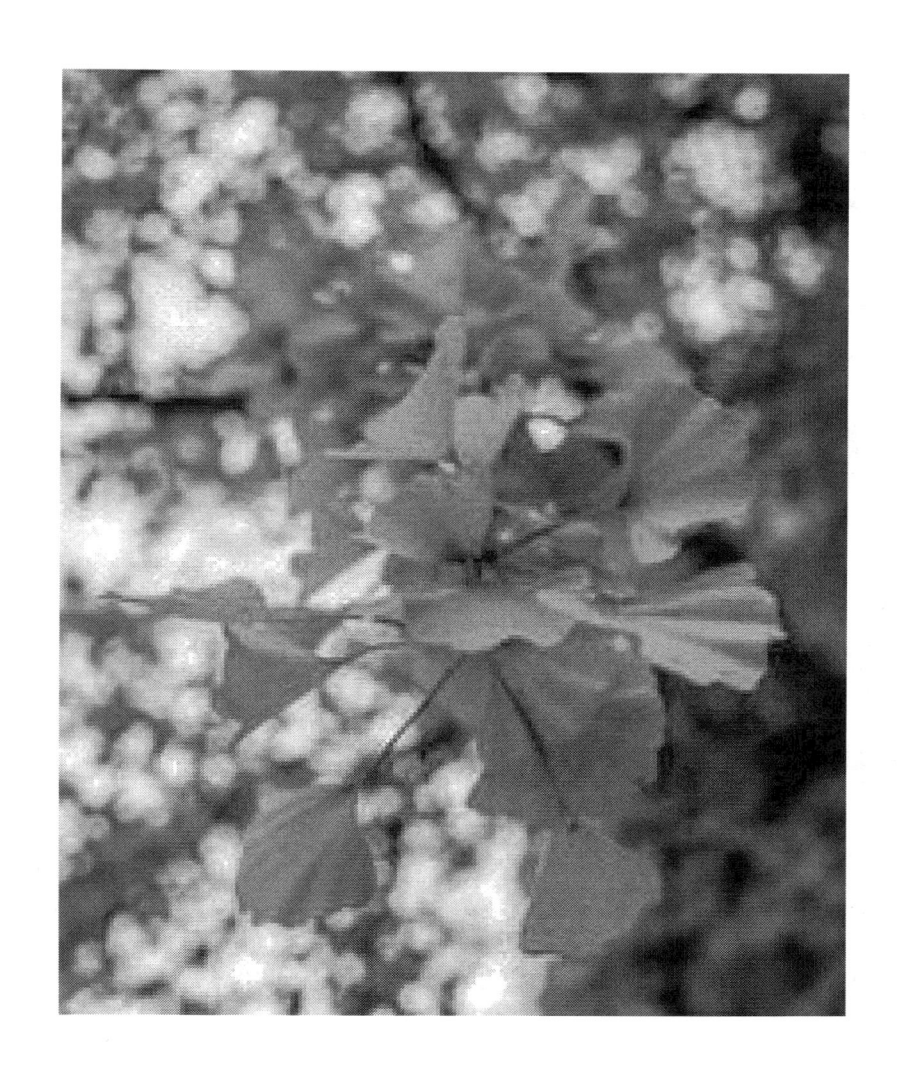

History of Ginkgo Plant

The Ginkgo tree, also known as Ginkgo biloba, is one of the oldest living tree species in the world. It is believed to have originated in China over 200 million years ago and has been cultivated and used for its medicinal properties for thousands of years. The tree is also considered a symbol of longevity, strength, and resilience, and it has been planted in many parks and gardens around the world as an ornamental tree. Ginkgo trees were nearly extinct at one point, but thanks to cultivation efforts, they are now widely available.

How to Grow Gingko

Ginkgo biloba is a tree commonly grown for its distinctive fan-shaped leaves and ornamental value. It is also known for its medicinal properties, particularly in improving cognitive function and circulation. Here are some tips on how to grow Ginkgo:

Climate: Ginkgo trees are hardy to USDA zones 3-8 and can tolerate a wide range of temperatures, from hot summers to cold winters. They prefer well-draining soil and full sun, but can also tolerate partial shade. Propagation: Ginkgo can be propagated from seeds, cuttings, or grafting. However, it's important to note that the seeds have a fleshy outer layer that can cause skin irritation, and they may take up to a year to germinate. Cuttings and grafting are faster methods of propagation.

Soil: Ginkgo trees prefer slightly acidic to neutral soil, with a pH between 5.0 and 7.5. They can tolerate different soil types, but do best in well-draining soils that are rich in organic matter.

Watering: Ginkgo trees have deep taproots and are relatively drought-tolerant, so they don't require frequent watering. However, they benefit from regular watering during hot and dry weather.

Pruning: Ginkgo trees have a naturally symmetrical shape and don't require much pruning. However, you can remove any dead or damaged branches in late winter or early spring.

Pests and Diseases: Ginkgo trees are generally resistant to pests and diseases, but can be affected by aphids, scale insects, and root rot in poorly draining soil.

By following these tips, you can successfully grow Ginkgo trees in your garden and enjoy their unique beauty and medicinal properties.

How to Clone Ginkgo Plant

Ginkgo trees can be propagated through both seeds and cuttings, but the success rate is higher with cuttings. Here are the steps to clone a ginkgo plant through cuttings:

Take cuttings: Collect cuttings from a healthy ginkgo tree during the dormant season in late winter or early spring. Choose a branch that is at least 1 year old and 1/4 to 1/2 inch in diameter. Cut a section of the branch that is 6 to 8 inches long, and make the cut just below a leaf node. Remove lower leaves: Remove all the leaves from the bottom half of the cutting, leaving only a few leaves at the top.

Dip in rooting hormone: Dip the cut end of the cutting in rooting hormone powder, which will help it to develop roots.

Plant in soil: Fill a container with well-draining potting soil, and poke a hole in the center with a pencil. Insert the cutting into the hole and gently press the soil around it.

Water and cover: Water the soil until it is moist, but not soggy. Cover the container with a clear plastic bag to create a mini greenhouse that will keep the cutting humid and warm.

Place in bright, indirect light: Place the container in a bright, warm spot that receives indirect sunlight. Avoid placing it in direct sunlight or in a drafty location.

Monitor and water regularly: Check the cutting daily to make sure the soil is still moist, and water as needed to keep it from drying out. After a few weeks, you should see new growth emerging from the top of the cutting, which is a sign that it has successfully rooted. You can remove the plastic bag at this point and gradually acclimate the plant to less humidity.

How is Ginkgo Plant Medicinal

Ginkgo is a popular herbal remedy that has been used for thousands of years in traditional Chinese medicine. The leaves of the Ginkgo biloba tree contain various compounds that are believed to have medicinal properties, such as flavonoids and terpenoids. Some of the potential health benefits associated with Ginkgo biloba include improving memory and cognitive function, reducing anxiety and depression, and improving circulation.

It is important to note that while there is some evidence to support the use of Ginkgo biloba for certain health conditions, more research is needed to fully understand its potential benefits and risks. As with any herbal remedy or supplement, it is recommended that individuals speak with their healthcare provider before use.

Medicinal Ginkgo Recipes

Ginkgo biloba, also known as maidenhair tree, is a popular herbal remedy in traditional medicine. The leaves of the ginkgo tree contain flavonoids and terpenoids, which are believed to have medicinal properties. Here are some medicinal ginkgo recipes:

Ginkgo tea: Steep dried ginkgo leaves in hot water for 5-10 minutes to make a refreshing and energizing tea. Ginkgo tea is said to improve cognitive function and boost memory.

Ginkgo tincture: To make a ginkgo tincture, place dried ginkgo leaves in a jar and cover with high-proof alcohol, such as vodka or brandy. Let the mixture sit for 4-6 weeks, shaking the jar every few days. Strain the liquid and store in a dark bottle. Take 1-2 droppers of the tincture in water as needed for improved circulation and brain function.

Ginkgo capsules: Ginkgo capsules are a convenient way to get the benefits of ginkgo on the go. Look for capsules that contain a standardized extract of ginkgo leaf, with at least 24% flavone glycosides and 6% terpene lactones. Take 120-240 mg per day for improved memory, focus, and circulation.

Ginkgo honey: Infuse honey with ginkgo leaf to make a sweet and medicinal treat. Heat honey in a double boiler and add dried ginkgo leaves. Let the mixture simmer for 20-30 minutes, stirring occasionally. Strain out the leaves and store the ginkgo honey in a jar. Take a spoonful of ginkgo honey as needed for improved cognitive function and immunity.

Ginseng

History of Ginseng

Ginseng is a popular herb used in traditional medicine practices throughout the world, particularly in Asia. The word ginseng comes from the Chinese term "rénshēn," which means "man root." This name reflects the appearance of the ginseng root, which resembles the shape of a human body. Ginseng has been used for centuries in traditional Chinese medicine to improve health and treat a wide range of medical conditions. It was also used in North America by indigenous peoples for its medicinal properties. Today, ginseng is still widely used in traditional medicine practices and is also used as a dietary supplement.

How to Grow Ginseng

Growing ginseng can be a challenging and time-consuming process, as this plant requires specific growing conditions to thrive. Here are some general steps to follow when growing ginseng:

Choose the right location: Ginseng prefers a shady location with well-draining soil that is rich in organic matter. The soil should have a pH of around 5.5 to 6.5.

Prepare the soil: The soil should be prepared in advance by removing any weeds, rocks, or other debris. The soil can be amended with organic matter, such as compost or leaf litter, to improve its quality.

Plant the seeds: Ginseng seeds are best planted in the fall, after the soil has cooled down but before it has frozen. The seeds should be planted about 1 inch deep and 4-6 inches apart. A light layer of mulch can be added on top to help retain moisture and regulate temperature.

Water and fertilize: Ginseng requires consistent moisture to grow properly, so be sure to water regularly, especially during dry spells. Fertilizer can also be added in the spring to help support growth.

Protect the plants: Ginseng is susceptible to damage from pests and diseases, so it's important to protect the plants with natural insecticides and fungicides as needed.

Harvest: Ginseng takes several years to mature, with the roots typically harvested after 5-6 years. To harvest, carefully dig up the roots, being careful not to damage them, and rinse them clean. The roots can be dried and used for medicinal purposes.

How to Clone Ginseng

Ginseng can be propagated through seeds, root cuttings, or tissue culture. However, it can take several years for the plants to mature enough to harvest the roots. Here are the steps for cloning ginseng using root cuttings:

Choose a healthy and mature ginseng plant that is at least 3 years old. Dig up the plant in the fall after the leaves have turned yellow and the plant has gone dormant.

Cut the roots into pieces that are about 2-3 inches long. Make sure each piece has at least one bud or "eye" and some small roots.

Plant the root cuttings in a well-draining potting mix that is slightly acidic (pH 5.5-6.5). Make a shallow trench in the soil and place the cutting horizontally with the bud facing up. Cover the cutting with soil, leaving the bud exposed.

Water the cutting thoroughly and keep the soil moist but not waterlogged. Place the pot in a shaded area that receives indirect sunlight. Keep the temperature around 70°F.

After a few weeks, you should see new growth emerging from the bud. Keep the soil moist and gradually increase the amount of sunlight the plant receives.

After a year or two, the ginseng plants should be mature enough to transplant to a permanent location outdoors.

How is Ginseng Medicinal

Ginseng is believed to have a wide range of health benefits and has been used in traditional medicine for centuries. Some of the reported medicinal properties of ginseng include:

Boosting the immune system: Ginseng is thought to have immune-boosting properties that can help fight off infections and diseases.

Reducing stress: Ginseng has been used to help reduce stress and anxiety, and may be helpful in managing depression.

Improving cognitive function: Some studies suggest that ginseng may help improve cognitive function, including memory and attention.

Lowering blood sugar: Ginseng may help regulate blood sugar levels and improve insulin sensitivity, making it potentially beneficial for people with diabetes.

Enhancing physical performance: Ginseng is believed to improve endurance, strength, and athletic performance.

Supporting heart health: Some research has suggested that ginseng may help lower blood pressure and reduce the risk of heart disease.

It's important to note that the research on the medicinal benefits of ginseng is still ongoing, and more studies are needed to confirm these reported health benefits. As with any herbal supplement or medication, it's important to talk to your healthcare provider before using ginseng to determine if it's safe and appropriate for you.

Medicinal Ginseng Recipes

Here are a few medicinal ginseng recipes:

Ginseng Tea: To make ginseng tea, steep 1 to 2 grams of ginseng root in hot water for 5 to 10 minutes. You can add a touch of honey or lemon juice to enhance the flavor. This tea is said to be energizing and can help to improve mental clarity.

Ginseng Chicken Soup: This recipe involves simmering a whole chicken with ginseng root and other ingredients like garlic, ginger, and jujube dates. The resulting soup is said to be nourishing and restorative.

Ginseng Tonic: To make a ginseng tonic, combine ginseng root with other herbs like astragalus, licorice root, and ginger. Steep the herbs in hot water for several hours or overnight, then strain and drink as a tonic. This is said to help support the immune system and promote overall vitality.

Ginseng Smoothie: Add a few slices of fresh or dried ginseng root to your favorite smoothie recipe for an energizing boost. Ginseng pairs well with berries, banana, and other tropical fruits.

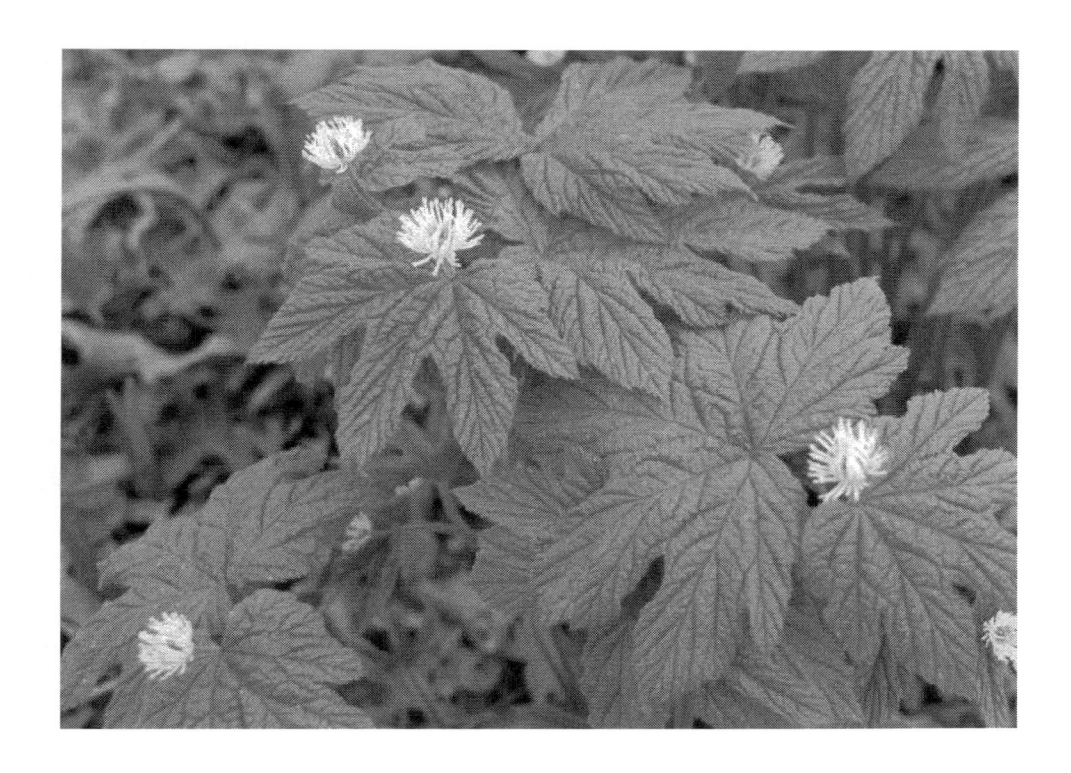

Goldenseal

History of Goldenseal

Goldenseal (Hydrastis canadensis) is a herbaceous perennial plant native to the eastern United States and southeastern Canada. The plant has been an important part of Native American medicine for centuries, and its use as a medicinal herb was later adopted by European settlers.

The Cherokee tribe used goldenseal for a variety of medicinal purposes, including as a treatment for inflammation, digestive issues, and infections. The Iroquois used goldenseal as a wash for sore eyes and as a treatment for colds, fevers, and digestive problems. They also used the plant as a dye for clothing and as a general tonic.

In the 19th century, goldenseal became popular in American medicine and was used to treat a range of ailments, including digestive issues, respiratory infections, and skin conditions. Today, the plant is still used as a natural remedy for various health conditions, although it is important to note that goldenseal has been overharvested and is now considered endangered in some areas.

How to Grow Goldenseal

Goldenseal is a perennial herb that is native to North America. It requires a moist, shady environment to thrive. Here are the steps to grow goldenseal:

Choose a location: Goldenseal should be grown in a shaded area with moist, well-drained soil. A woodland or a shaded area with partial sun is ideal.

Prepare the soil: Goldenseal prefers a slightly acidic soil pH (around 6.0). You can amend the soil with organic matter such as compost or leaf mold to improve drainage and fertility.

Plant the goldenseal: Plant goldenseal in the spring or fall. The roots should be planted about 2 inches deep, with a spacing of 6-8 inches between plants. The crown of the root should be slightly above the soil level.

Water regularly: Keep the soil consistently moist, but not waterlogged.

Water the goldenseal regularly, especially during dry periods.

Mulch: Apply a layer of organic mulch such as shredded leaves or straw around the plants to help retain moisture and control weeds.

Harvest: Goldenseal roots can be harvested after 3-4 years of growth. Only harvest a small portion of the roots at a time, leaving the majority in the ground to ensure the plant continues to thrive.

Note: Goldenseal is a threatened plant species in the wild and should only be grown and harvested sustainably. It is important to purchase goldenseal seeds or plants from reputable sources and avoid harvesting wild populations.

How to Clone Goldenseal

Goldenseal (Hydrastis canadensis) can be propagated through rhizome division or seed. Here are the steps for cloning goldenseal through rhizome division:

Dig up the mature goldenseal plant in the fall after the foliage has died back.

Use a sharp, clean knife to carefully divide the rhizomes into sections, making sure each section has at least one bud and some roots attached. Plant the divided rhizomes immediately in a shady, moist spot with well-draining soil.

Water the newly planted rhizomes thoroughly and keep the soil consistently moist until new growth appears.

Mulch around the plants with a layer of leaf litter or straw to help retain moisture and regulate temperature.

It's important to note that goldenseal is a slow-growing plant and can take several years to establish, so patience is key when growing this herb.

How is Goldenseal Medicinal

Goldenseal is a popular medicinal herb with a long history of use in traditional medicine. The root and rhizome (underground stem) of the goldenseal plant contain several active compounds, including berberine, hydrastine, and canadine, which are believed to have various health benefits. Here are some of the medicinal uses of goldenseal:

Immune system support: Goldenseal is believed to have immune-boosting properties, which can help the body fight off infections and illnesses. Digestive health: Goldenseal has been used to improve digestive health, relieve diarrhea and constipation, and promote overall gastrointestinal health.

Respiratory health: Goldenseal is used to treat respiratory infections and congestion, including colds, flu, and sinusitis.

Skin health: Goldenseal has been used topically to treat skin infections, wounds, and rashes.

Anti-inflammatory: Goldenseal has been used to reduce inflammation and relieve pain, including in cases of arthritis and other inflammatory conditions.

It is important to note that goldenseal should be used under the guidance of a healthcare professional, as it can interact with certain medications and may have side effects in some people.

Medicinal Goldenseal Recipes

Goldenseal is a medicinal herb that has been traditionally used to treat various ailments, including digestive problems, respiratory infections, and skin conditions. Here are a few medicinal Goldenseal recipes:

Goldenseal Tea: Take a teaspoon of dried Goldenseal root powder and add it to a cup of hot water. Let it steep for 10-15 minutes and strain the tea. You can drink this tea twice a day to alleviate digestive issues and respiratory infections.

Goldenseal Tincture: Take 1-2 ounces of dried Goldenseal root and chop it finely. Place the chopped root in a jar and cover it with 80-100 proof vodka. Seal the jar and shake it every day for 2-3 weeks. After the tincture is ready, strain it and store it in a dark glass bottle. You can take 1-2 drops of this tincture in a glass of water up to three times a day to treat infections and boost immunity.

Goldenseal Salve: Melt one cup of coconut oil in a double boiler and add 1/4 cup of dried Goldenseal root powder. Heat the mixture for 30 minutes, stirring frequently. Strain the mixture through a cheesecloth and let it cool. Once the mixture has cooled, add 10-15 drops of tea tree oil and stir well.

Transfer the mixture to a glass jar and store it in a cool, dark place. You can apply this salve topically to treat skin infections, rashes, and minor wounds.

Holy Basil

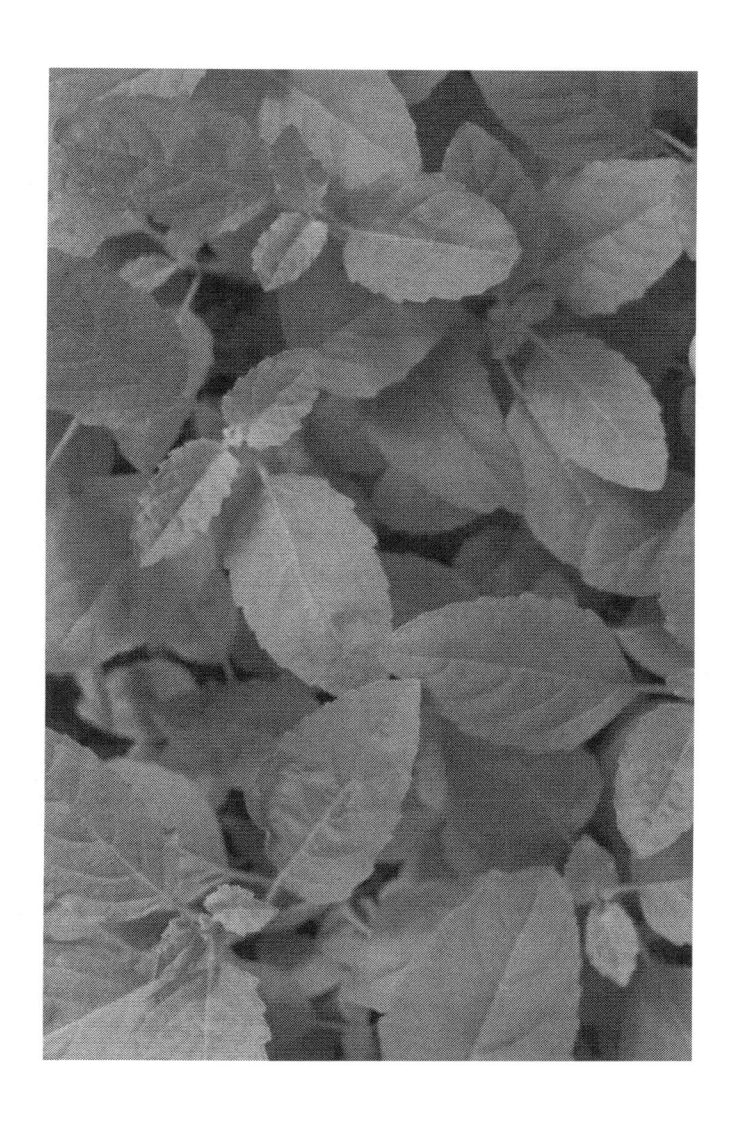

History of Holy Basil

Holy basil, also known as Tulsi, has a rich history in Ayurvedic medicine and Indian culture. Here are some key historical points:

Ancient India: Holy basil has been cultivated in India for over 3,000 years and has been used in Ayurvedic medicine to treat a variety of ailments, including respiratory infections, fever, and digestive issues.

Hinduism: Holy basil is considered a sacred plant in Hinduism and is often planted around temples and homes. It is believed to have spiritual and medicinal properties, and is used in daily rituals and ceremonies.

Greek and Roman medicine: Holy basil was introduced to the Mediterranean region by the Greeks and Romans, who used it for its medicinal properties.

World War II: During World War II, holy basil was used as an antidote to the effects of radiation exposure.

Modern research: In recent years, modern research has confirmed many of the traditional uses of holy basil. Studies have shown that holy basil has anti-inflammatory, anti-anxiety, and anti-diabetic properties, and may be effective in treating a variety of health conditions.

Today, holy basil is widely cultivated and used around the world for its medicinal properties and as a culinary herb. It is available in various forms, including teas, tinctures, and supplements.

How to Grow Holy Basil

Here are the steps to grow holy basil, also known as Tulsi:

Choose a location: Holy basil is a warm-weather plant that requires full sunlight and well-drained soil. Choose a location that receives at least 6 hours of direct sunlight each day and has well-drained soil.

Prepare the soil: Holy basil grows best in soil that is slightly acidic with a pH between 6.0 and 7.5. Work compost or well-rotted manure into the soil to improve fertility and drainage.

Sow the seeds: Sow the holy basil seeds directly in the garden bed, about ¼ inch deep and 10-12 inches apart. Alternatively, you can start the seeds indoors in small pots, 4-6 weeks before the last frost date.

Water the seeds: Water the seeds immediately after planting and keep the soil moist until the seedlings emerge. Once the seedlings have emerged, water them deeply once a week.

Thin the seedlings: When the seedlings are about 2-3 inches tall, thin them to one plant every 10-12 inches. This will give each plant enough space to grow and produce a good crop.

Fertilize: Holy basil is a heavy feeder and requires regular fertilization. You can use a balanced fertilizer or a fertilizer high in nitrogen to promote leaf growth.

Harvest: Holy basil can be harvested once the plant has grown to about 6 inches tall. Pinch off the leaves and stems as needed, being careful not to remove more than one-third of the plant at a time.

Overwinter: If you live in a region with mild winters, holy basil may survive outdoors through the winter. However, if you live in a colder climate, you may want to dig up the plant and overwinter it indoors.

With proper care, holy basil can grow to be a tall, bushy plant that produces abundant leaves and flowers. It is a relatively easy plant to grow, making it a great choice for beginner gardeners.

How to Clone Holy Basil Tulsi Plant

Here are the steps to clone a holy basil (Tulsi) plant:

Choose a healthy Tulsi plant: Select a healthy Tulsi plant with vibrant green leaves and no signs of disease or pests.

Take a cutting: Use a clean, sharp pair of scissors or garden shears to cut a stem from the Tulsi plant that is about 4-6 inches long. Cut the stem at a 45-degree angle just below a node, which is where a leaf is attached to the stem.

Remove the lower leaves: Carefully remove the lower leaves from the stem, leaving only the top few leaves intact.

Dip the stem in rooting hormone: Dip the cut end of the stem in rooting hormone powder, which can be purchased at a garden center or online. This will help to stimulate root growth.

Plant the cutting: Plant the stem in a pot filled with moist potting soil, making sure to bury the node where the leaves were removed. Gently press the soil around the stem to hold it in place.

Water the cutting: Water the cutting thoroughly, making sure the soil is moist but not waterlogged.

Cover the cutting: Cover the cutting with a clear plastic bag to create a humid environment that will help the cutting to root. Place the pot in a warm, bright location, but out of direct sunlight.

Monitor the cutting: Check the cutting regularly to make sure the soil is moist and that the plastic bag is not too wet or too dry. After a few weeks, the cutting should begin to develop roots.

Remove the plastic bag: Once the cutting has developed roots, remove the plastic bag and continue to care for the plant as you would a mature Tulsi plant.

Note: You can also clone Tulsi plants using water propagation or air layering methods.

How is Holy Basil Medicinal

Holy basil, also known as Tulsi, has been used for centuries in Ayurvedic medicine to treat a wide range of health conditions. Here are some of the medicinal properties and benefits of holy basil:

Anti-inflammatory: Holy basil contains compounds that have anti-inflammatory properties, which may help to reduce inflammation and pain in the body.

Anti-anxiety: Holy basil has been shown to have anti-anxiety properties, and may help to reduce stress and promote relaxation.

Antioxidant: Holy basil is rich in antioxidants, which help to protect the body from damage caused by free radicals and may help to prevent chronic diseases.

Immune-boosting: Holy basil has immune-boosting properties, and may help to strengthen the immune system and protect against infections. Anti-diabetic: Holy basil has been shown to help regulate blood sugar levels in people with diabetes, and may be beneficial for people with insulin resistance.

Cardiovascular health: Holy basil may help to lower cholesterol levels and improve cardiovascular health.

Respiratory health: Holy basil has been traditionally used to treat respiratory infections, and may be beneficial for people with asthma or chronic obstructive pulmonary disease (COPD).

Holy basil can be consumed in various forms, including teas, tinctures, and supplements. It is generally considered safe, but as with any supplement, it is important to speak with a healthcare provider before taking it, particularly if you are pregnant or taking medications.

Medicinal Recipes for Holy Basil

Holy basil, also known as Tulsi, has a long history of use in Ayurvedic medicine for its medicinal properties. Here are some medicinal recipes that use holy basil:

Tulsi tea: Add a few fresh Tulsi leaves to a cup of hot water and steep for several minutes. This tea is said to help with respiratory issues, stress, and anxiety.

Tulsi juice: Blend a handful of Tulsi leaves with water to create a juice. This juice can be used to treat coughs, colds, and other respiratory issues. Tulsi paste: Crush a handful of fresh Tulsi leaves to create a paste. Apply this paste to the forehead to relieve headaches or to the chest to help with respiratory issues.

Tulsi honey: Mix a handful of Tulsi leaves with a cup of honey. This mixture can be taken daily to boost the immune system and provide relief from respiratory issues.

Tulsi oil: Infuse Tulsi leaves in coconut or sesame oil for several days to create a medicinal oil that can be used for massages, to relieve joint pain and inflammation, and to promote relaxation.

Tulsi tincture: Steep a handful of Tulsi leaves in vodka or another high-proof alcohol for several weeks to create a tincture. This tincture can be taken orally to boost the immune system, promote relaxation, and provide relief from digestive issues.

These are just a few examples of the many ways in which Tulsi can be used medicinally. As with any herbal remedy, it is important to consult with a healthcare provider before using Tulsi for medicinal purposes, particularly if you are pregnant or taking medications.

Lavender

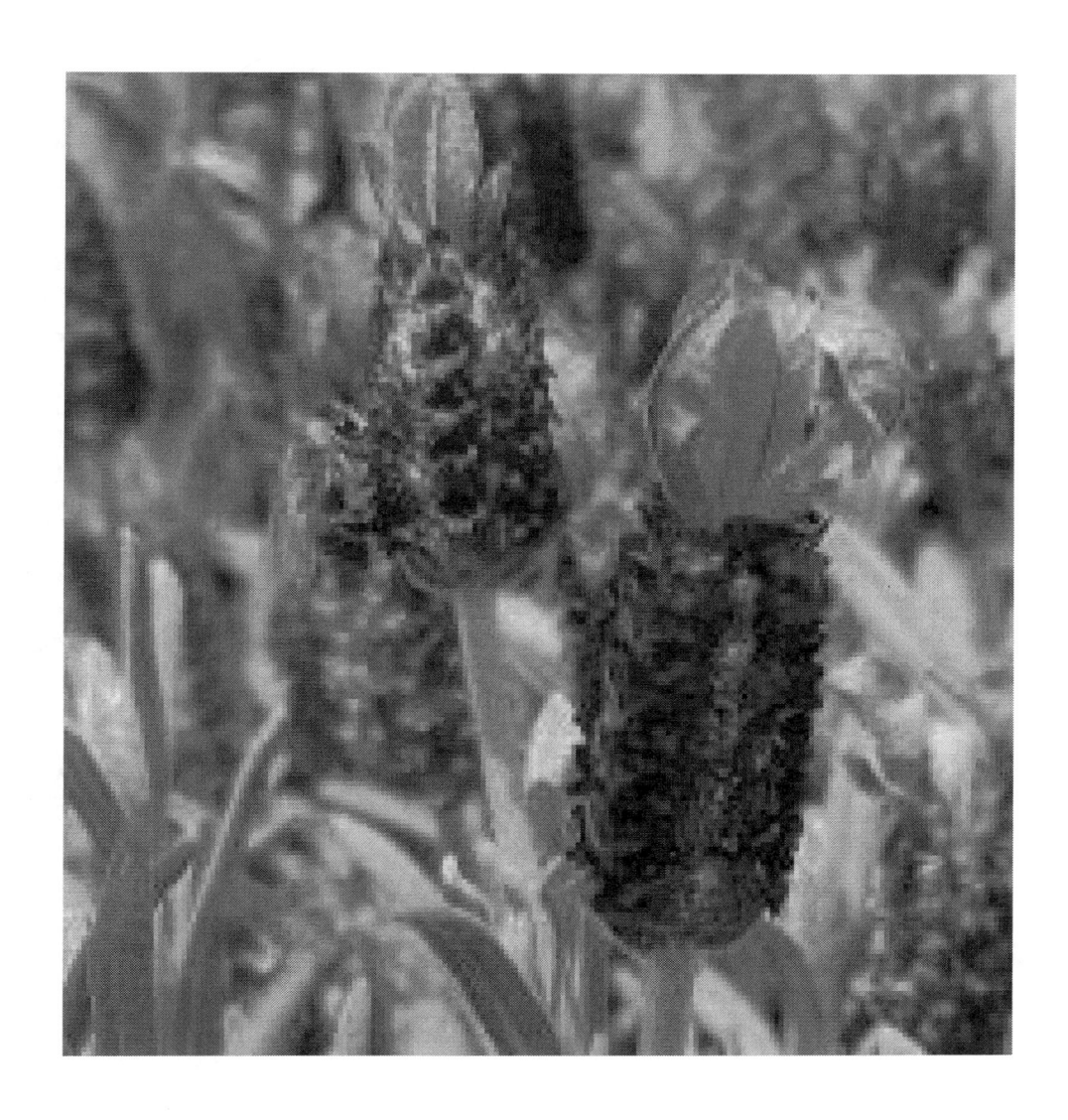

History of Lavender Plant

Lavender (Lavandula) has a long and rich history dating back thousands of years. Here are some key historical facts about the lavender plant:

Lavender is believed to have originated in the Mediterranean region, specifically in the mountainous areas of the western Mediterranean. Ancient Egyptians used lavender in their mummification process, as well as for perfumes and cosmetics.

In ancient Greece, lavender was used to scent baths and as a perfume for clothing and linens.

The Romans used lavender for medicinal purposes, such as treating wounds and digestive issues. They also used it in their baths and for perfumes.

During the Middle Ages, lavender was grown in monastic gardens and used for medicinal and culinary purposes. It was believed to have a calming effect on the body and mind.

Lavender became popular in the 17th and 18th centuries in Europe as a fragrance for soaps, cosmetics, and perfumes. It was also used to scent linens and repel moths.

In the 19th century, lavender became popular in the United Kingdom for its medicinal properties, particularly for treating headaches and respiratory issues.

Today, lavender is still widely used for its soothing and relaxing properties. It is used in aromatherapy, skincare, and culinary applications.

Overall, lavender has a rich history and has been valued for its fragrance and medicinal properties for thousands of years.

How to Grow Lavender

Lavender (Lavandula) is a popular herb that is known for its fragrant flowers and soothing properties. Here are some steps to help you grow lavender:

Choose the right variety: Lavender comes in many different varieties, so choose one that is suited to your climate and growing conditions. Some popular varieties include English lavender (Lavandula angustifolia), French lavender (Lavandula stoechas), and Spanish lavender (Lavandula dentata). Plant in the right location: Lavender prefers full sun and well-drained soil. Choose a location that receives at least 6 hours of sunlight per day and has soil that is slightly alkaline and well-drained. If your soil is heavy clay, consider amending it with sand or other materials to improve drainage. Plant at the right time: Lavender can be planted in the spring or fall, but it's best to avoid planting in the hottest part of the summer. If you're planting from seed, start indoors about 6-8 weeks before the last frost date in your area.

Space the plants: Lavender plants should be spaced about 12-18 inches apart, depending on the variety. This will allow the plants to have enough room to grow and prevent overcrowding.

Water regularly: Lavender plants prefer to be kept on the dry side, so don't overwater. Water deeply once a week, or when the soil is dry to the touch. Avoid getting water on the foliage, as this can promote fungal diseases.

Prune regularly: Lavender should be pruned regularly to maintain its shape and promote bushier growth. Prune back about one-third of the plant after it has finished flowering in the summer. You can also prune lightly in the spring to remove any dead or damaged growth.

By following these steps, you should be able to successfully grow lavender and enjoy its beautiful fragrance and calming properties.

How to Clone Lavender Plant

Lavender can be propagated by taking cuttings from an established plant. Here are some steps to help you clone lavender:

Choose a healthy plant: Select a healthy lavender plant with no signs of disease or damage. Choose a stem that is firm and woody, not soft and green.

Take a cutting: Use a sharp, clean pair of pruning shears to take a cutting from the plant. Cut a stem that is about 4-6 inches long, just below a leaf node.

Remove the lower leaves: Strip the lower leaves from the stem, leaving only a few at the top. This will help the cutting focus its energy on growing roots, rather than supporting leaves.

Dip in rooting hormone: Dip the cut end of the stem into rooting hormone powder. This will help promote root growth.

Plant in potting mix: Plant the cutting in a pot filled with well-draining potting mix. Water the soil lightly, but avoid getting water on the leaves.

Cover and mist: Cover the pot with a plastic bag or plastic wrap to create a humid environment. Mist the cutting regularly to keep the soil moist and encourage root growth.

Wait for roots to grow: It can take several weeks for roots to grow, so be patient. Check the cutting periodically by gently tugging on it to see if it has rooted. Once the cutting has rooted, you can remove the plastic covering and transplant the lavender into a larger pot or into your garden.

By following these steps, you should be able to successfully clone lavender and enjoy its fragrant blooms in your garden.

How is Lavender Medicinal

Lavender has many medicinal properties and has been used for centuries for its health benefits. Here are some of the ways that lavender is used medicinally:

Relaxation and sleep: Lavender is known for its calming and relaxing properties. It has been shown to help reduce anxiety and promote sleep, making it a popular natural remedy for insomnia.

Pain relief: Lavender has anti-inflammatory properties and can help relieve pain and swelling. It is often used to treat headaches, muscle aches, and joint pain.

Skin health: Lavender has antiseptic and anti-inflammatory properties that make it useful for treating skin conditions like acne, eczema, and psoriasis. It can also help soothe sunburns and insect bites.

Respiratory health: Lavender can help relieve respiratory issues like coughs and colds. It has been shown to have expectorant properties, which can help loosen mucus and make it easier to breathe.

Digestive health: Lavender can help promote digestive health by soothing the stomach and reducing inflammation. It can also help relieve symptoms of irritable bowel syndrome (IBS) and other digestive disorders.

Lavender is typically used in the form of essential oil, which can be applied topically or diffused into the air. It can also be consumed in tea or supplement form. However, it is important to note that lavender should be used with caution and under the guidance of a healthcare professional, as it can interact with certain medications and may cause allergic reactions in some people.

Medicinal Recipes with Lavender

Here are some medicinal recipes that use lavender:

Lavender tea: Steep 2 teaspoons of dried lavender flowers in hot water for 5-10 minutes. Strain and drink to promote relaxation, relieve anxiety, and aid in digestion.

Lavender oil massage blend: Mix 10 drops of lavender essential oil with 1 tablespoon of carrier oil (such as sweet almond oil or coconut oil). Use this blend to massage sore muscles and joints, relieve headaches, and promote relaxation.

Lavender inhalation: Add a few drops of lavender essential oil to a bowl of hot water. Lean over the bowl with a towel over your head and inhale deeply for a few minutes to relieve respiratory issues like coughs and colds. Lavender bath salts: Mix 1 cup of Epsom salt, 1/2 cup of sea salt, and 10 drops of lavender essential oil in a bowl. Add the mixture to a warm bath and soak for 20-30 minutes to soothe sore muscles, promote relaxation, and relieve stress.

Lavender and honey cough syrup: Mix 1 tablespoon of dried lavender flowers with 1 cup of boiling water. Steep for 15-20 minutes, then strain. Mix the lavender tea with 1/4 cup of honey and 1 tablespoon of lemon juice. Take 1-2 teaspoons as needed to relieve coughs and soothe sore throats. It is important to note that while lavender is generally safe for most people, it can cause allergic reactions in some individuals. If you experience any adverse reactions, stop using lavender immediately and consult with a healthcare professional.

Lemongrass

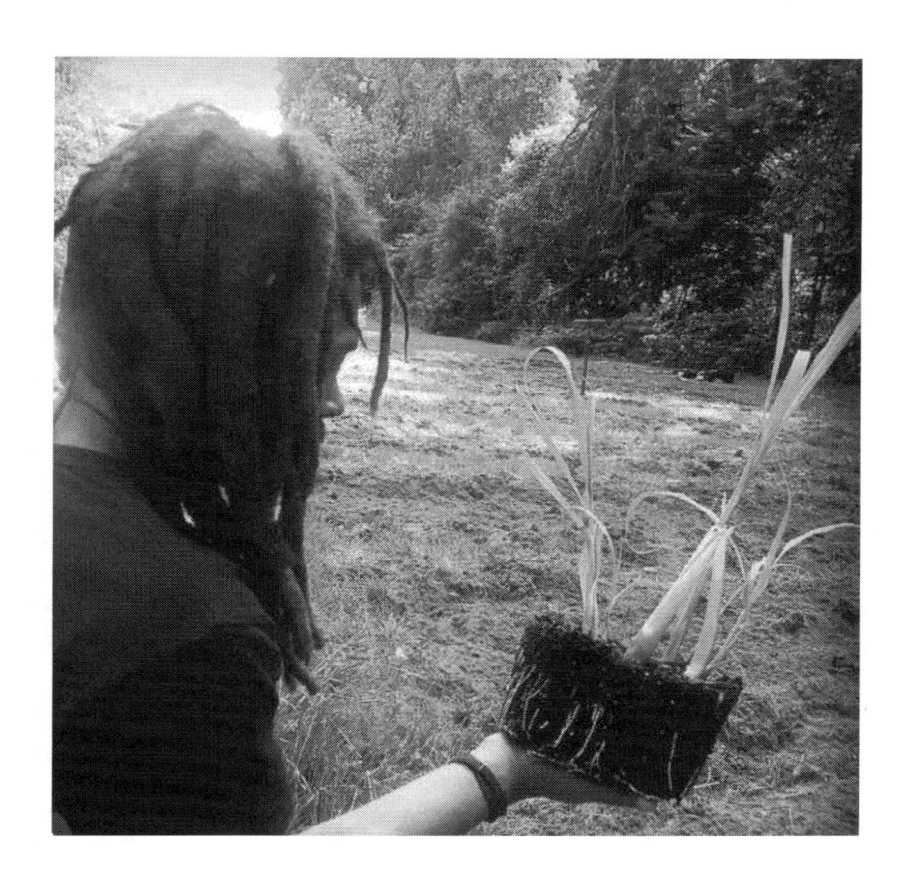

History of Lemongrass

Lemongrass (Cymbopogon citratus) is a herbaceous plant native to tropical regions of Asia and Africa. It has been used for medicinal and culinary purposes for centuries. It is believed to have originated in India, where it was used for cooking, as a tea, and for medicinal purposes. Lemongrass was introduced to the rest of the world through the spice trade and is now widely cultivated in many countries, including Thailand, Malaysia, and the United States. It is commonly used in Southeast Asian cuisines, as well as in teas, essential oils, and other products for its aromatic and medicinal properties.

How to Grow Lemongrass

Lemongrass is a tropical plant that is commonly used in Asian cuisine and is also known for its medicinal properties. Here are the steps to grow lemongrass:

Choosing a Location: Lemongrass requires plenty of sunlight and warmth, so choose a spot that receives at least 6 hours of direct sunlight and is protected from cold drafts.

Soil Preparation: Lemongrass grows well in well-drained soil that is rich in organic matter. Before planting, amend the soil with compost or well-rotted manure to improve soil fertility.

Planting: You can start growing lemongrass from seeds, but it's much easier to propagate it from mature plants. Simply buy a few stalks of fresh lemongrass from the grocery store or a nursery and trim off the bottom 2-3 inches of the stalks. Place them in a glass of water and wait until roots start to emerge. Once the roots are about 2 inches long, plant the lemongrass in the soil, spacing the plants about 3 feet apart.

Watering: Lemongrass requires regular watering to keep the soil moist, especially during the hot summer months. Water deeply once or twice a week, or more frequently if the soil is drying out quickly.

Fertilizing: Feed the lemongrass with a balanced fertilizer once a month during the growing season.

Harvesting: You can start harvesting lemongrass when the stalks are about a foot tall. Simply cut the stalks at the base and use the tender lower portion for cooking or making tea.

Winter Care: Lemongrass is not frost-tolerant, so if you live in a colder climate, you'll need to protect the plants from freezing temperatures. You can either dig up the plants and grow them indoors over the winter or cover them with a thick layer of mulch to insulate the roots.

How is Lemongrass Medicinal

Lemongrass is a herb that has been used for centuries in traditional medicine to treat various ailments. It contains several beneficial compounds, including citral, which gives it its characteristic lemony scent and flavor. The following are some of the medicinal properties and uses of lemongrass:

Digestive health: Lemongrass has been traditionally used to improve digestion, alleviate stomach problems such as bloating and constipation, and stimulate bowel movements.

Pain relief: Lemongrass oil has anti-inflammatory and analgesic properties, which can help relieve pain caused by conditions such as arthritis, muscle soreness, and headaches.

Respiratory health: Lemongrass has antibacterial and antifungal properties, which make it useful for treating respiratory infections, such as colds, coughs, and bronchitis.

Stress and anxiety relief: Lemongrass contains compounds that have a calming effect on the mind and body, which can help reduce stress, anxiety, and promote relaxation.

Skin health: Lemongrass oil has antiseptic and astringent properties, which can help treat skin infections, acne, and oily skin.

Insect repellent: Lemongrass oil is a natural insect repellent and can be used to repel mosquitoes and other insects.

Overall, lemongrass is a versatile herb with many potential health benefits. However, it is important to note that more research is needed to fully understand its medicinal properties and potential side effects.

Medicinal Lemongrass Recipes

Lemongrass is a popular herb used in cooking, but it also has medicinal properties. Here are a few recipes that use lemongrass for its health benefits:

Lemongrass tea: Boil a few stalks of lemongrass in water and let it steep for a few minutes. Add honey and lemon juice to taste. This tea can help with digestion, relieve anxiety, and boost the immune system.

Lemongrass essential oil massage: Mix a few drops of lemongrass essential oil with a carrier oil like coconut oil and use it for a relaxing massage. Lemongrass oil is known to have anti-inflammatory and pain-relieving properties, making it a great choice for massage.

Lemongrass soup: Lemongrass is a common ingredient in soups, especially in Southeast Asian cuisine. Combine lemongrass with other herbs and spices like ginger and turmeric for a delicious and healthy soup that can help with cold and flu symptoms.

Lemongrass bath soak: Add a few drops of lemongrass essential oil to your bathwater for a relaxing and invigorating soak. The scent of lemongrass is known to reduce stress and anxiety, while also providing a refreshing fragrance.

Rosemary

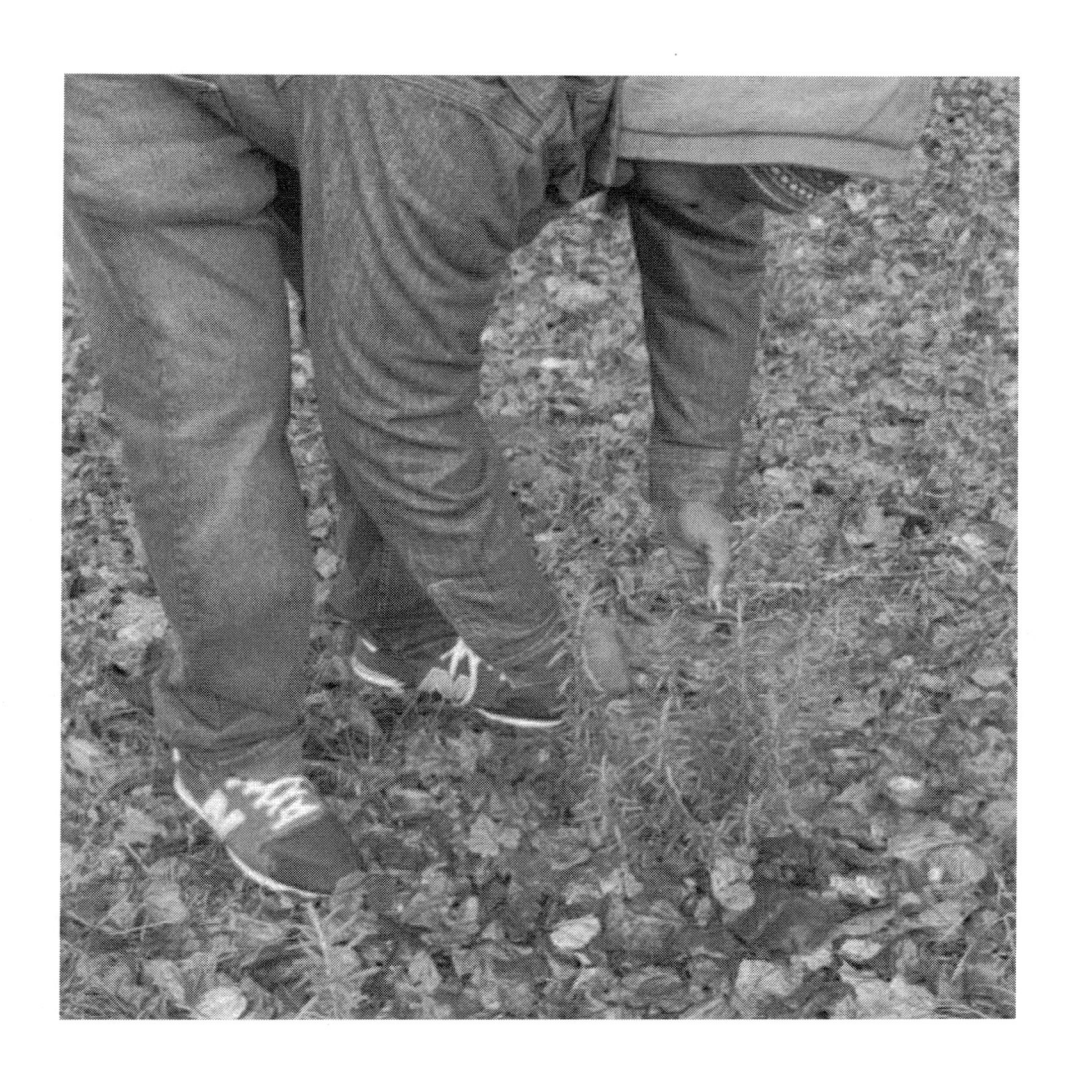

History of Rosemary Plant

Rosemary (Rosmarinus officinalis) is a woody, perennial herb that has been cultivated and used for thousands of years. The plant is native to the Mediterranean region, but is now widely grown throughout the world.

Rosemary has a rich history and has been used for a variety of purposes. In ancient Greece and Rome, the herb was believed to improve memory and was often used in religious ceremonies. The Greek physician Dioscorides recommended rosemary for a variety of ailments, including indigestion and headaches.

During the Middle Ages, rosemary was used as a symbol of fidelity and was often included in wedding ceremonies. The herb was also used to ward off evil spirits and protect against the plague.

In addition to its medicinal and symbolic uses, rosemary has long been used in cooking. The herb is a popular seasoning for meats, vegetables, and breads, and is a key ingredient in many traditional Mediterranean dishes.

Today, rosemary continues to be valued for its medicinal, culinary, and aromatic properties. It is also used in cosmetics and perfumes, and is a popular ingredient in aromatherapy and herbal medicine.

How to Grow Rosemary

Rosemary is a woody, perennial herb with fragrant, needle-like leaves. Here are the steps to grow rosemary:

Choose a location: Rosemary prefers full sun and well-drained soil. Choose a location that receives at least 6 hours of direct sunlight per day.

Planting: Plant your rosemary in the spring, after the last frost. You can grow rosemary from seeds, cuttings or purchased seedlings. If planting from seed, sow the seeds indoors about 8-10 weeks before the last frost. Soil preparation: Prepare the soil by adding organic matter, such as compost, to improve drainage and fertility. Rosemary prefers soil with a pH of 6.0-7.0.

Watering: Water your rosemary regularly, but do not overwater. Allow the soil to dry out between watering to prevent root rot. Rosemary is drought-tolerant and does not require frequent watering.

Fertilizing: Fertilize your rosemary with a balanced fertilizer in the spring and mid-summer. Do not over-fertilize, as this can cause the plant to produce more foliage than essential oils.

Pruning: Prune your rosemary regularly to maintain its shape and promote bushy growth. You can also prune to harvest the leaves for culinary use. Harvesting: Harvest the leaves as needed throughout the growing season. Rosemary leaves are most flavorful when harvested before the plant flowers.

With these tips, you should be able to successfully grow rosemary in your garden or indoor herb garden.

How to Clone Rosemary Plant

Rosemary can be easily propagated by taking stem cuttings from a healthy, mature plant. Here are the steps to clone a rosemary plant:

Choose a stem: Choose a healthy stem from a mature rosemary plant that is at least 6 inches long and has several sets of leaves.

Cut the stem: Use a clean, sharp pair of pruning shears to cut the stem at a 45-degree angle, just below a node where a leaf meets the stem.

Remove lower leaves: Remove the leaves from the bottom 2 inches of the stem. This will be the part of the stem that will be inserted into the soil. Dip in rooting hormone: Dip the cut end of the stem in rooting hormone powder, which will encourage the stem to produce roots.

Plant the stem: Insert the stem into a pot filled with moist potting soil. Make a hole in the soil with a pencil or chopstick and gently insert the stem into the hole.

Cover with plastic: Cover the pot with a plastic bag or clear plastic wrap to create a mini greenhouse. This will help keep the soil moist and humid, which will encourage rooting.

Place in a bright, warm location: Place the pot in a bright, warm location, but out of direct sunlight. Keep the soil moist but not waterlogged.

Wait for roots to form: Check the stem after a few weeks to see if roots have formed. You can gently tug on the stem to see if it resists, which indicates that roots have formed.

Transplant: Once the stem has formed roots, transplant it into a larger pot or into your garden.

With these steps, you should be able to successfully clone a rosemary plant and grow a new, healthy plant.

How is Rosemary Medicinal

Rosemary has a long history of medicinal use and has been traditionally used for a wide range of ailments. Here are some of the medicinal benefits of rosemary:

Anti-inflammatory: Rosemary contains compounds that have anti-inflammatory properties, making it useful in the treatment of conditions such as arthritis, asthma, and other inflammatory diseases.

Digestive aid: Rosemary has been used as a digestive aid for centuries. It can help stimulate digestion, relieve constipation, and reduce gas and bloating.

Memory enhancer: Rosemary has been traditionally used to enhance memory and cognitive function. Research suggests that the herb may help improve concentration, mental clarity, and memory retention.

Pain reliever: Rosemary has analgesic properties and may help relieve pain from headaches, menstrual cramps, and other types of pain. Immune booster: Rosemary contains antioxidants and other compounds that may help boost the immune system and protect against infections. Stress reliever: Rosemary has a calming effect on the nervous system and may help reduce stress and anxiety.

Rosemary can be used in a variety of forms, including teas, tinctures, essential oils, and capsules. However, it's important to note that while rosemary has many potential health benefits, it should not be used as a substitute for medical treatment or as a replacement for prescribed medications without consulting a healthcare professional.

Medicinal Recipes with Rosemary

Rosemary is a versatile herb that can be used in a variety of medicinal recipes. Here are a few recipes to try:

Rosemary tea for digestion: Steep a handful of fresh rosemary sprigs in hot water for 10-15 minutes. Strain and sweeten with honey, if desired. Drink this tea after a meal to help stimulate digestion and relieve digestive discomfort.

Rosemary and lavender bath salts for relaxation: Mix together 1 cup of Epsom salt, 1/2 cup of sea salt, 1/4 cup of dried rosemary leaves, and 1/4 cup of dried lavender flowers. Add a few drops of rosemary and lavender essential oils, if desired. Add 1/2 cup of the mixture to a warm bath and soak for 20-30 minutes to relax and soothe sore muscles.

Rosemary and honey cough syrup: Simmer 1 cup of fresh rosemary leaves in 2 cups of water for 30 minutes. Strain and add 1 cup of honey. Simmer for an additional 10-15 minutes until the mixture has thickened. Store in a glass jar and take 1-2 teaspoons as needed to relieve cough and sore throat.

Rosemary and olive oil scalp treatment: Mix together 1/2 cup of olive oil and 1/4 cup of fresh rosemary leaves in a small saucepan. Heat over low heat for 10-15 minutes until the oil is infused with the rosemary scent. Let cool and strain the oil. Massage the oil into your scalp and hair, cover with a shower cap, and leave on for 30 minutes before shampooing. This treatment can help stimulate hair growth and relieve scalp irritation.

These are just a few examples of the many ways you can use rosemary for medicinal purposes. As always, it's important to consult a healthcare professional before using any herbs or natural remedies to ensure they are safe for you to use.

Sage

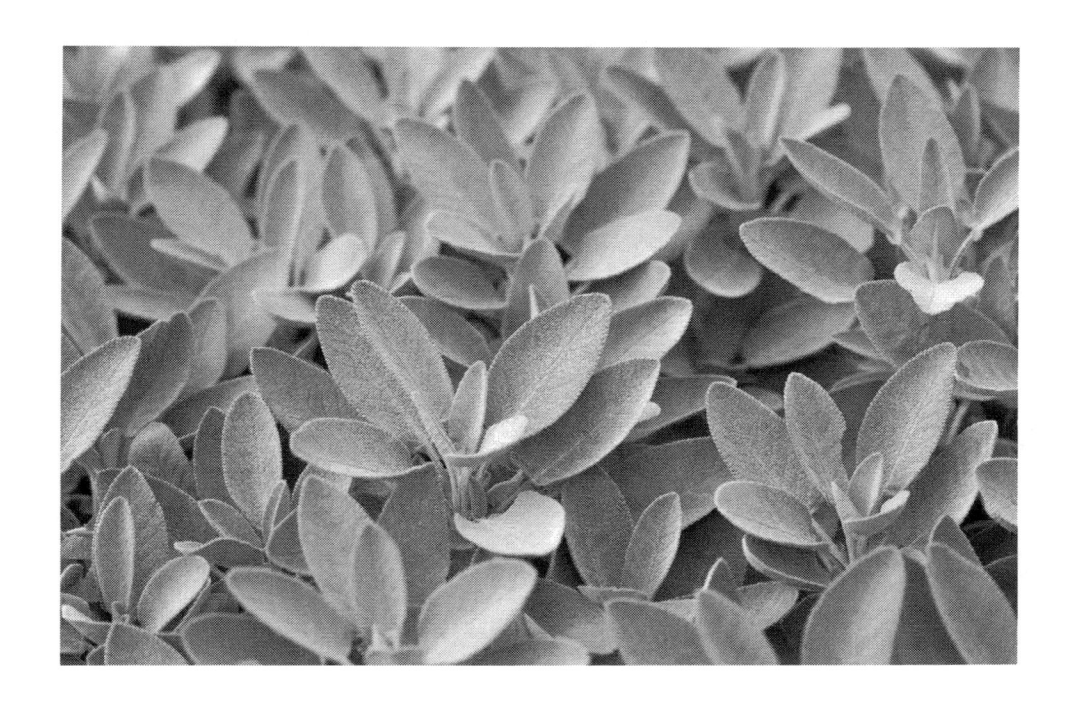

History of Sage Plant

Sage (Salvia officinalis) has a long history of use as a medicinal herb and culinary spice. It is native to the Mediterranean region and has been cultivated for thousands of years.

The ancient Greeks and Romans revered sage for its healing properties, and it was considered a sacred herb in many cultures. In medieval Europe, it was believed to have the power to ward off evil spirits, and it was often used in ceremonies and rituals.

Sage was also used for culinary purposes, both for flavoring food and as a preservative. It was commonly used to flavor meats, soups, and stews, and was also used to make tea and other beverages.

Today, sage is still widely used as a culinary herb, and is also used in a variety of herbal remedies. It is believed to have anti-inflammatory, antioxidant, and antimicrobial properties, and is often used to relieve digestive problems, soothe sore throats, and treat skin conditions.

Overall, sage has a rich and fascinating history, and its versatility and numerous health benefits continue to make it a popular herb today.

How to Grow Sage

Sage is a relatively easy herb to grow and care for. Here are the steps to grow sage:

Choose a location: Sage thrives in full sun and well-draining soil. Choose a location in your garden that gets at least 6-8 hours of sunlight per day and has soil that drains well.

Plant seeds or seedlings: Sage can be grown from seeds or seedlings. If starting from seeds, sow them 1/4 inch deep in the soil and keep the soil moist until the seeds germinate. If starting from seedlings, dig a hole in the soil that is slightly larger than the root ball of the seedling and gently place the seedling in the hole. Water thoroughly after planting.

Water regularly: Sage prefers soil that is kept consistently moist but not waterlogged. Water deeply once a week or as needed to keep the soil evenly moist.

Fertilize sparingly: Sage doesn't require a lot of fertilizer. You can add a slow-release fertilizer to the soil at the time of planting, or fertilize sparingly with a balanced fertilizer once or twice during the growing season.

Prune regularly: Pruning sage regularly can help keep the plant bushy and prevent it from becoming woody. Pinch off the tips of the branches when they are about 6-8 inches long, and prune the plant back by 1/3 in the spring.

Harvest leaves as needed: Sage leaves can be harvested as needed once the plant is established. Pinch off individual leaves or cut off entire branches, leaving at least two sets of leaves on the stem.

By following these steps, you should be able to grow a healthy and productive sage plant that will provide you with flavorful leaves for cooking or for making tea.

How to Clone Sage Plant

Sage (Salvia officinalis) is a perennial herb that can be easily propagated through stem cuttings. Here are the steps to clone a sage plant:

Choose a stem: Look for a stem that is healthy and free from disease. The stem should be at least 4-6 inches long and have several sets of leaves. Cut the stem: Use clean, sharp scissors or pruning shears to cut the stem at a 45-degree angle, just below a node (where the leaves attach to the stem). Remove the leaves from the lower half of the stem.

Prepare the cutting: Dip the cut end of the stem in rooting hormone powder to help it develop roots. Shake off any excess powder.

Plant the cutting: Fill a small pot with a well-draining soil mix, such as a mixture of perlite and peat moss. Make a small hole in the soil with a pencil or your finger, and gently insert the cut end of the stem into the hole. Firm the soil around the stem to hold it in place.

Water the cutting: Water the cutting thoroughly to settle the soil and moisten the stem. Be sure not to overwater, as this can cause the cutting to rot. Keep the soil moist but not waterlogged.

Provide the right conditions: Place the pot in a warm, bright location, but out of direct sunlight. Cover the pot with a plastic bag or a clear plastic container to create a humid environment for the cutting.

Wait for roots to develop: Check the cutting after a few weeks to see if roots have developed. Gently tug on the stem to feel for resistance, which indicates that the cutting has rooted. Once the cutting has rooted, you can remove the plastic covering and care for the plant as you would a mature sage plant.

By following these steps, you should be able to clone your sage plant and grow a new plant from a stem cutting.

How is Sage Medicinal

Sage (Salvia officinalis) is a medicinal herb that has been used for thousands of years for its various health benefits. Here are some of the ways sage is believed to be medicinal:

Anti-inflammatory: Sage contains compounds that have anti-inflammatory properties, which may help reduce inflammation throughout the body. Antimicrobial: Sage has natural antimicrobial properties that may help fight off harmful bacteria, viruses, and fungi.

Antioxidant: Sage is high in antioxidants, which can help protect the body against oxidative stress and reduce the risk of chronic diseases. Digestive aid: Sage is believed to have a soothing effect on the digestive system, and may help relieve digestive discomfort such as gas, bloating, and constipation.

Memory and cognitive function: Sage has been traditionally used to enhance memory and cognitive function. Some studies have suggested that sage may help improve memory and attention in older adults. Menopausal symptoms: Sage is believed to have estrogenic properties, which may help alleviate symptoms of menopause such as hot flashes and night sweats.

Sage can be used in a variety of ways to reap its medicinal benefits. It can be brewed into a tea, used as a seasoning in cooking, or taken in supplement form. As with any herbal remedy, it's important to consult a healthcare professional before using sage for medicinal purposes to ensure it is safe and appropriate for you.

Medicinal Recipes with Sage

Sage (Salvia officinalis) is a versatile herb that can be used in a variety of medicinal recipes. Here are a few examples:

Sage tea: To make sage tea, steep a few fresh or dried sage leaves in hot water for 5-10 minutes. This tea can be enjoyed as a digestive aid or for its antimicrobial and anti-inflammatory properties.

Sage-infused oil: To make sage-infused oil, place a handful of fresh sage leaves in a jar and cover with olive oil. Let the mixture sit for 2-4 weeks, shaking the jar daily. Strain the oil and use it topically for its anti-inflammatory and antimicrobial properties.

Sage honey: To make sage honey, place a few fresh sage leaves in a jar and cover with honey. Let the mixture sit for 1-2 weeks, stirring occasionally. Strain the honey and use it to soothe sore throats or as a natural sweetener.

Sage steam inhalation: To make a sage steam inhalation, add a handful of fresh or dried sage leaves to a pot of boiling water. Cover your head with a towel and inhale the steam for 5-10 minutes. This can help relieve congestion and respiratory infections.

Sage mouthwash:

Ingredients:

- 1 cup of water
- 2 tablespoons of dried sage leaves
- 1 teaspoon of sea salt or Himalayan salt
- Optional: 2-3 drops of peppermint essential oil (for added freshness)

Instructions:

1. Boil the water in a saucepan.
2. Once the water has come to a boil, remove it from heat and add the dried sage leaves.
3. Cover the saucepan and let the sage leaves steep in the hot water for about 15-20 minutes.
4. After the steeping time, strain the liquid using a fine-mesh sieve or cheesecloth to remove the sage leaves. Allow the liquid to cool.
5. Once the liquid has cooled, add the sea salt or Himalayan salt to the mixture and stir until it dissolves completely.
6. If desired, add a few drops of peppermint essential oil for a refreshing flavor.
7. Transfer the mouthwash into a clean, sterilized glass bottle or jar with a tight-fitting lid.
8. Your sage mouthwash is now ready to use.

To use the sage mouthwash:

1. Shake the bottle well before each use to ensure the ingredients are mixed.
2. Take a small amount of the mouthwash (about 1/4 to 1/2 cup) into your mouth.
3. Swish the mouthwash around in your mouth for about 30-60 seconds, making sure to reach all areas of your mouth, including between the teeth and along the gums.

4. Spit out the mouthwash into the sink.

5. Rinse your mouth with water to remove any residual mouthwash.

6. Use the sage mouthwash once or twice daily, or as needed.

Sage is known for its antimicrobial and astringent properties, which can help promote oral health and freshen breath. However, if you have any underlying dental or oral health conditions, it's always a good idea to consult with a dentist or healthcare professional before using homemade mouthwash.

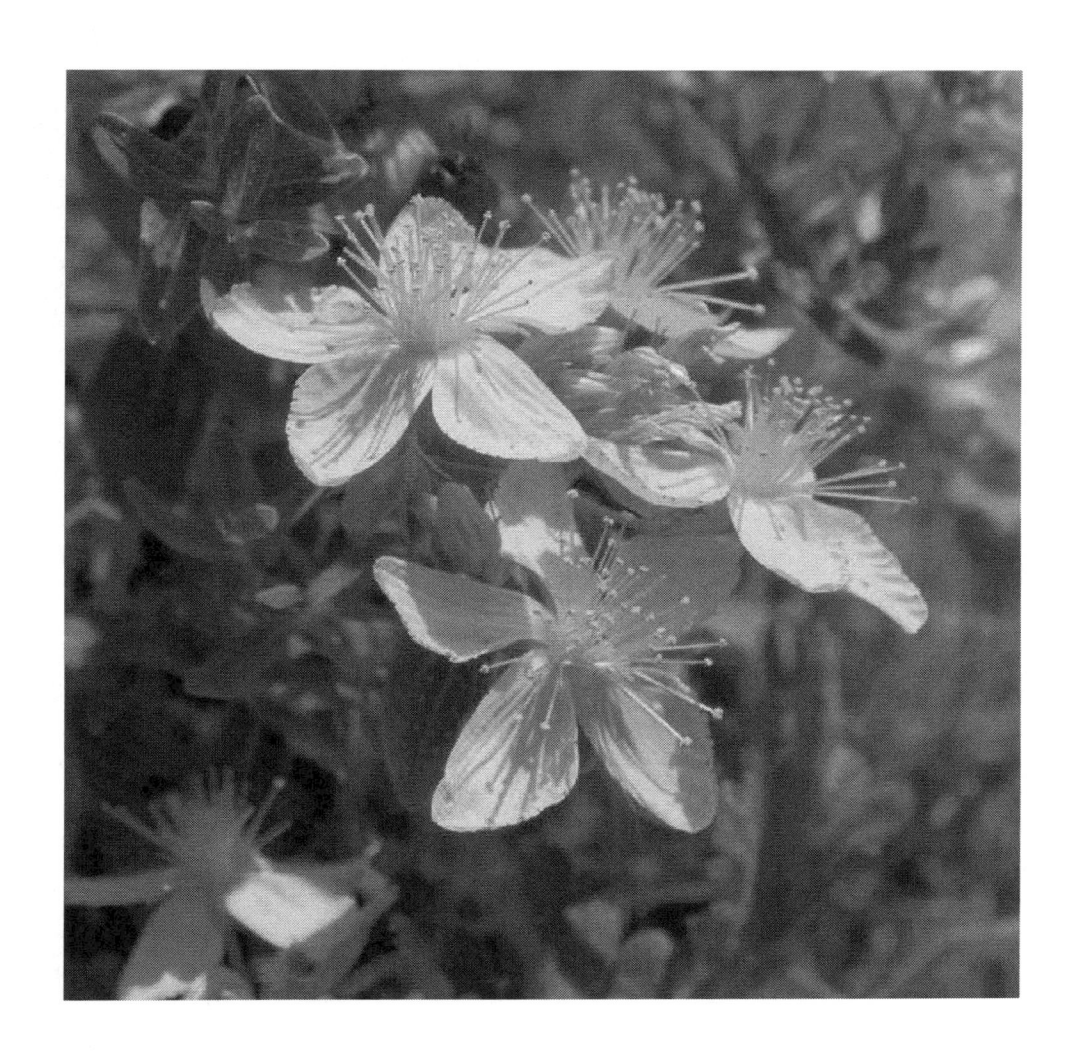

Saint John's Wort

History of Saint John's Wort

Saint John's wort, also known as Hypericum perforatum, has a long history of use as a medicinal herb. The plant is native to Europe but has also been naturalized in North America, Asia, and Australia.

The use of St. John's wort as a medicinal herb can be traced back to the ancient Greeks. The physician Hippocrates, known as the "Father of Medicine," recommended it for a variety of conditions, including nerve pain and inflammation. Later, the Roman naturalist Pliny the Elder also wrote about the medicinal properties of St. John's wort.

In the Middle Ages, St. John's wort was believed to have powerful healing properties and was used to treat a range of ailments, including wounds, burns, and nervous disorders. The herb was also believed to have protective properties and was used to ward off evil spirits.

In more recent times, St. John's wort has been extensively studied for its potential use in treating depression and anxiety. The herb has also been used to treat other conditions, including nerve pain, inflammation, and viral infections.

How to Grow Saint John's Wort

Here are some general tips for growing St. John's wort:

Location: St. John's wort prefers full sun to partial shade, and well-draining soil. It can tolerate different soil types, but it prefers a slightly acidic to neutral pH. Choose a spot that gets at least 6 hours of direct sunlight each day.

Planting: You can plant St. John's wort seeds directly in the garden in early spring, or you can start them indoors 6-8 weeks before the last frost date. Plant the seeds 1/4 inch deep and space them 12-18 inches apart. Water well after planting.

Watering: St. John's wort prefers well-draining soil, so make sure not to overwater it. Water deeply once a week, or more often if the soil feels dry to the touch.

Fertilizing: St. John's wort doesn't require much fertilizer, but you can give it a boost with a balanced fertilizer once a month during the growing season. Pruning: St. John's wort can grow up to 3 feet tall and wide, so it's a good idea to prune it in late winter or early spring to promote bushy growth. Cut back any dead or damaged branches, and shape the plant to your desired size.

Pests and Diseases: St. John's wort is relatively pest-free, but it can be susceptible to root rot if the soil is too wet. Make sure the soil has good drainage, and avoid overwatering.

How to Clone Saint John's Wort

St. John's wort can be propagated through stem cuttings. Here's how to clone St. John's wort:

Select a healthy stem: Choose a stem from the St. John's wort plant that is at least 6 inches long and has several sets of leaves.

Cut the stem: Use a sharp, clean pair of scissors or pruning shears to cut the stem just below a set of leaves. Make the cut at a 45-degree angle. Strip the leaves: Remove the leaves from the lower half of the stem.

Dip in rooting hormone: Dip the cut end of the stem in rooting hormone powder or gel. This will help the cutting to develop roots.

Plant the cutting: Fill a small pot with well-draining potting soil. Make a hole in the soil with your finger, and insert the cut end of the stem into the hole. Gently press the soil around the stem to hold it in place.

Water the cutting: Water the cutting thoroughly, and place the pot in a bright, but not direct sunlight. Keep the soil moist but not waterlogged. Wait for roots to develop: In about 3-4 weeks, the cutting should start to develop roots. You can check by gently tugging on the stem. If you feel resistance, the roots have formed.

Transplant the cutting: Once the roots are well established, you can transplant the St. John's wort cutting into a larger pot or directly into the garden.

How is Saint John's Wort Medicinal

Saint John's wort has been traditionally used for a variety of medicinal purposes, including:

Depression and anxiety: St. John's wort has been studied info extensively for its use in treating mild to moderate depression and anxiety. The herb is thought to work by increasing levels of serotonin, dopamine, and norepinephrine in the brain.

Nerve pain: St. John's wort has been used to treat nerve pain and neuralgia, particularly when it is associated with shingles or other viral infections.

Wound healing: St. John's wort has been used topically to promote wound healing and to reduce inflammation and pain associated with burns, cuts, and other skin injuries.

Menopausal symptoms: St. John's wort has been used to reduce the frequency and severity of hot flashes and other menopausal symptoms. Seasonal affective disorder (SAD): St. John's wort has been used to treat SAD, a type of depression that occurs during the winter months.

It is important to note that St. John's wort can interact with certain medications, including antidepressants, birth control pills, and blood thinners. It is important to speak with a healthcare provider before using St. John's wort for any medicinal purposes.

Medicinal Saint John's Wort Recipes

Saint John's wort can be used in various forms for its medicinal properties. Here are a few recipes:

Saint John's wort tea: Steep 1-2 teaspoons of dried Saint John's wort flowers in a cup of hot water for 10-15 minutes. Strain and drink the tea 1-2 times a day. This tea is commonly used for anxiety and depression.

Saint John's wort oil: Combine dried Saint John's wort flowers with olive oil or another carrier oil in a glass jar. Let the mixture sit in a sunny spot for several weeks, shaking the jar daily. Strain the oil and store it in a dark glass bottle. This oil can be used topically to reduce inflammation and pain associated with burns, cuts, and other skin injuries.

Saint John's wort tincture: Combine fresh or dried Saint John's wort flowers with vodka or another high-proof alcohol in a glass jar. Let the mixture sit for several weeks, shaking the jar daily. Strain the liquid and store it in a dark glass bottle. This tincture can be used to treat depression, anxiety, and nerve pain.

It is important to note that the dosage and preparation of Saint John's wort can vary depending on the intended use and individual factors such as age and health status. It is recommended to consult with a healthcare provider before using Saint John's wort for medicinal purposes.

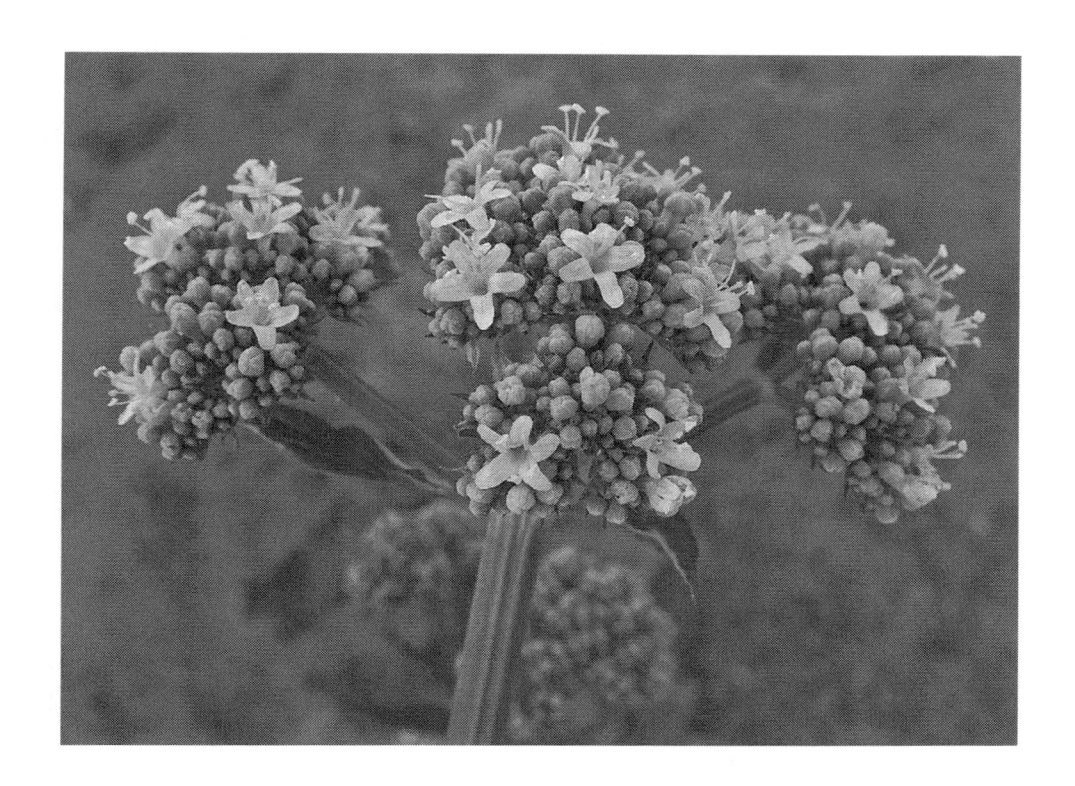

Valerian Root

History of Valerian Plant

Valerian (Valeriana officinalis) has a long history of use as a medicinal herb. Its use dates back to ancient Greece and Rome, where it was believed to have sedative and calming properties. The Greek physician Hippocrates recommended it for insomnia, and the Roman naturalist Pliny the Elder described its use as a diuretic, digestive aid, and treatment for headaches and nervousness.

In medieval Europe, Valerian became popular as a treatment for a variety of ailments, including anxiety, epilepsy, and digestive problems. It was also used as a flavoring agent in food and beverages, and was believed to have aphrodisiac properties.

Valerian continued to be used as a medicinal herb in the centuries that followed, and was brought to North America by European settlers. Today, Valerian is still used as a natural remedy for insomnia, anxiety, and other nervous system disorders. Its active compounds, valerenic acid and valeranone, are believed to have sedative and anxiolytic effects, and research has shown that Valerian can be an effective treatment for mild to moderate insomnia.

How to Grow Valerian Root

Here are the steps to grow Valerian root:

Choose a planting site: Valerian root grows best in well-drained soil that is rich in organic matter. The site should receive partial shade to full sun. Prepare the soil: Work the soil to a depth of 12-18 inches, removing any weeds or debris. Add compost or well-rotted manure to the soil to improve its texture and fertility.

Plant the seeds or root cuttings: Valerian can be grown from seeds or root cuttings. If planting seeds, sow them in the soil in early spring or fall. Cover the seeds with a light layer of soil and water them regularly. If using root cuttings, plant them in the soil in early spring or fall, burying them about 2 inches deep.

Water and fertilize: Keep the soil moist, but not waterlogged. Fertilize the plants with a balanced fertilizer in the spring and mid-summer.

Harvest the root: The root of the Valerian plant is typically harvested in the fall of the second year. Carefully dig up the roots and wash them thoroughly. The roots can be dried and used for medicinal purposes. Valerian can grow up to 5 feet tall and can spread quickly, so be sure to plant it in an area where it has room to grow. Additionally, the plant has a strong odor that some people may find unpleasant, so it is best planted away from living areas.

How to Clone Valerian

Valerian can be propagated through root division or stem cuttings. Here are the steps for each method:

Root division: In the fall of the second year, when the roots are ready for harvest, dig up the plant carefully. Wash the roots and cut them into pieces that are 3-4 inches long. Each piece should have a bud or shoot attached to it. Plant the cuttings in well-draining soil, burying them about 2 inches deep. Keep the soil moist but not waterlogged, and place the cuttings in a partially shaded area until they start to develop new growth.

Stem cuttings: Take cuttings from healthy, mature Valerian plants in the spring or summer when the plant is actively growing. Cut a 6-inch long stem from the plant, just below a leaf node. Remove the lower leaves from the stem, leaving just a few leaves at the top. Dip the cut end in rooting hormone and plant the cutting in well-draining soil, burying it about 2 inches deep. Keep the soil moist and place the cutting in a partially shaded area until it starts to develop new growth.

It is important to note that Valerian can be a bit difficult to propagate, and not all cuttings will successfully root. Be patient and persistent, and you should eventually be able to successfully clone your Valerian plants.

How is Valerian Medicinal

Valerian (Valeriana officinalis) is commonly used as a natural remedy for insomnia, anxiety, and other nervous system disorders. Its active compounds, valerenic acid and valeranone, are believed to have sedative and anxiolytic effects, and research has shown that Valerian can be an effective treatment for mild to moderate insomnia.

Valerian is also used as a natural remedy for anxiety, stress, and nervous tension. Some studies have found that Valerian may be as effective as benzodiazepines, a class of drugs commonly used to treat anxiety disorders, but with fewer side effects.

Other potential medicinal uses of Valerian include as a treatment for menstrual cramps, muscle and joint pain, and headaches. It may also have anti-inflammatory and antioxidant properties, and some studies suggest that it may help improve cognitive function and memory.

It's worth noting that while Valerian is generally considered safe when used as directed, it can cause side effects in some people, including headaches, dizziness, upset stomach, and drowsiness. It may also interact with certain medications, so it's important to talk to a healthcare professional before using Valerian as a natural remedy.

Medicinal Valerian Recipes

Valerian root is commonly consumed as a tea or in supplement form as a natural remedy for insomnia, anxiety, and other nervous system disorders. Here are a few recipes that use Valerian:

Valerian Tea:

Steep 1-2 teaspoons of dried Valerian root in a cup of hot water for 10-15 minutes.

Strain the mixture and drink it before bedtime for a calming effect.

Sleepytime Tea:

Mix together 1 tablespoon of dried Valerian root, 1 tablespoon of dried chamomile flowers, and 1 tablespoon of dried passionflower. Steep the mixture in a cup of hot water for 10-15 minutes.

Strain the mixture and drink it before bedtime for a relaxing and calming effect.

Valerian Tincture:

Mix 1 part dried Valerian root with 5 parts 80 proof alcohol (such as vodka) in a jar with a tight-fitting lid.

Shake the jar daily for 2-3 weeks.

Strain the mixture and store the tincture in a dark glass bottle.

Take 1-2 dropperfuls (about 20-40 drops) in a small amount of water before bedtime for a calming and sedative effect.

It's important to note that Valerian root can cause drowsiness, so it should only be taken before bedtime or when you don't need to be alert or operate heavy machinery. Additionally, it's important to talk to a healthcare professional before using Valerian as a natural remedy, especially if you're pregnant, breastfeeding, or taking any medications.

Valerian Root recipe

Here is a simple recipe for valerian root tea:

Ingredients:

- 1 teaspoon dried valerian root
- 1 cup boiling water

Instructions:

Place the dried valerian root in a teapot or a mug.

Pour boiling water over the valerian root.

Cover the pot or mug and let steep for 10-15 minutes.

Strain the tea into another cup and discard the valerian root.

Sweeten with honey or stevia if desired.

Drink the tea 30 minutes to an hour before bedtime for a calming effect. Note: Valerian root can have a strong and somewhat unpleasant smell, but the tea itself has a milder taste. If you prefer a stronger tea, you can increase the amount of valerian root used. It is always recommended to consult with a healthcare professional before using valerian root or any other herbal supplement.

Witch Hazel

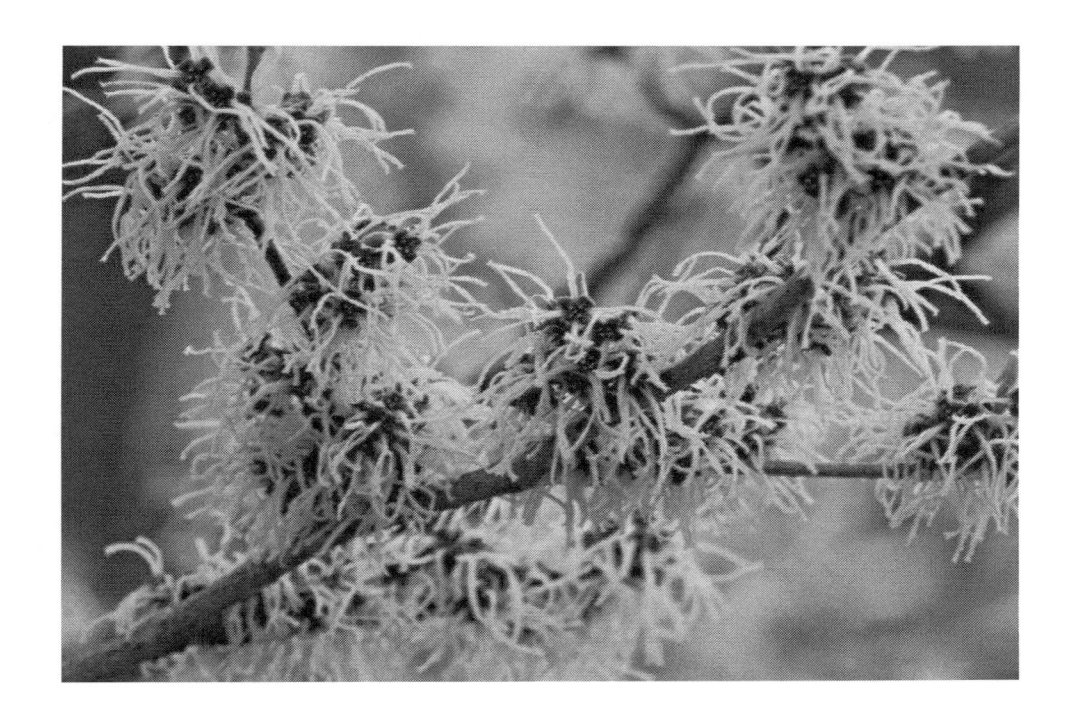

History of Witch Hazel

Witch hazel (Hamamelis virginiana) is a flowering shrub that is native to North America. The plant has a long history of use by indigenous peoples, who used it for a variety of medicinal purposes, including as a topical treatment for skin irritations, wounds, and hemorrhoids.

The name "witch hazel" comes from the Middle English word "wiche," which means "pliant" or "bendable," and the Old English word "wice," which means "willow." The plant was given this name because of its pliant, flexible branches, which were used by early settlers to create divining rods.

In the early 19th century, witch hazel extract became a popular natural remedy in the United States, and it was included in the United States Pharmacopeia as a topical treatment for a variety of skin conditions. Today, witch hazel is still widely used as a natural remedy for skin irritations and other conditions. It is also commonly used as an ingredient in natural skincare products.

How to Grow Witch Hazel

Witch hazel (Hamamelis virginiana) is a shrub or small tree that is native to North America. It is known for its attractive flowers and leaves, and its medicinal properties. Here are some general tips for growing witch hazel:

Choose the right location: Witch hazel prefers a partially shaded location with well-draining soil that is slightly acidic. It can tolerate full sun, but may suffer from leaf scorch in hot, dry weather.

Plant in the fall: The best time to plant witch hazel is in the fall, after the leaves have fallen off the tree. This will give the plant time to establish itself before the hot summer weather arrives.

Water regularly: Witch hazel prefers consistently moist soil, so be sure to water it regularly, especially during hot, dry weather.

Mulch around the base: Adding a layer of mulch around the base of the plant will help retain moisture and regulate soil temperature.

Prune after flowering: Witch hazel blooms in late winter to early spring, before the leaves emerge. Prune it after flowering, if needed, to maintain its shape and remove any dead or damaged wood.

As for cloning witch hazel, it can be propagated through softwood cuttings taken in early summer or hardwood cuttings taken in the fall.

How to Clone Witch Hazel

Witch hazel can be propagated through both softwood and hardwood cuttings. Here's how to clone witch hazel using the softwood cutting method:

Take softwood cuttings: Softwood cuttings are taken from the tips of the branches during the growing season. Cut a 4-6 inch long stem that is flexible, green, and has a few leaves on it.

Remove the leaves: Remove the leaves from the bottom 2/3 of the cutting, leaving a few leaves at the top.

Dip in rooting hormone: Dip the cut end of the stem in rooting hormone to encourage root development.

Plant the cutting: Fill a container with moist potting soil and make a hole in the center with a pencil. Insert the cutting in the hole, and gently press the soil around the stem.

Cover the container: Cover the container with a clear plastic bag, creating a mini greenhouse to trap moisture.

Provide bright, indirect light: Place the container in bright, indirect light, but avoid direct sunlight.

Water regularly: Keep the soil moist but not waterlogged. Water the cutting regularly, but do not overwater.

Monitor for roots: After a few weeks, gently tug on the cutting to see if it has rooted. Once roots have developed, you can transplant the cutting into a larger pot or into the ground.

Note: Hardwood cuttings are taken in late fall or winter when the leaves have fallen off the plant. The process is similar to the softwood method, but the cuttings will need to be stored in a cool, dark place until the following spring before planting.

How is Witch Hazel Medicinal?

Witch hazel has been used for medicinal purposes for centuries. The bark, leaves, and twigs of the witch hazel plant contain tannins and volatile oils that have astringent, anti-inflammatory, and antioxidant properties. These properties make it useful for a variety of skin conditions, including:

Acne: The astringent properties of witch hazel help to tighten the skin and reduce inflammation, making it effective in treating acne.

Eczema: Witch hazel can help reduce inflammation and itching associated with eczema. Its antioxidant properties also help to protect the skin from damage caused by free radicals.

Sunburn: Applying witch hazel to sunburned skin can help to soothe the burn and reduce inflammation.

Hemorrhoids: Witch hazel can be used topically to help reduce swelling and inflammation associated with hemorrhoids.

Minor cuts and bruises: Witch hazel has been used for centuries as a natural remedy for minor cuts and bruises due to its astringent and anti-inflammatory properties.

Varicose veins: Witch hazel can be used topically to help reduce swelling and inflammation associated with varicose veins.

Insect bites and stings: Witch hazel can help to reduce the itching and inflammation associated with insect bites and stings.

Overall, witch hazel is a versatile and effective natural remedy for a variety of skin conditions.

Medicinal Witch Hazel Recipes

Witch hazel has astringent and anti-inflammatory properties, making it useful in treating a variety of skin conditions such as acne, eczema, psoriasis, and insect bites. Here are some medicinal recipes using witch hazel:

Witch Hazel Toner: Witch hazel can be used as a natural toner to cleanse and tighten pores. Combine 1/2 cup witch hazel extract, 1/4 cup distilled water, and 10 drops of essential oil of your choice (such as lavender or tea tree). Store in a clean bottle and apply with a cotton pad after cleansing your face.

Soothing Face Mist: Combine 1/4 cup witch hazel extract, 1/4 cup rose water, and 1 tablespoon aloe vera gel in a spray bottle. Shake well and mist over your face as needed for a refreshing and soothing effect.

Hemorrhoid Relief: Witch hazel can be used to treat hemorrhoids due to its anti-inflammatory properties. Soak a cotton pad in witch hazel extract and apply it to the affected area for relief.

Scalp Treatment: Witch hazel can also be used to treat itchy and irritated scalp. Mix 1/4 cup witch hazel extract, 1/4 cup apple cider vinegar, and 10 drops of essential oil of your choice (such as peppermint or rosemary).

Apply to your scalp and let it sit for 10-15 minutes before shampooing as usual.

Sunburn Relief: Witch hazel can help soothe sunburned skin. Mix 1/2 cup witch hazel extract, 1/4 cup aloe vera gel, and 10 drops of lavender essential oil. Apply to the affected area for relief.

Infections & Medicinal Plants That May Help

Medicinal herbs can potentially help with various types of infections, but it's important to note that their effectiveness may vary, and they should not replace medical treatment. Here are some infections for which medicinal herbs are commonly used as complementary or supportive remedies:

Dental infections: Clove oil (Syzygium aromaticum) is often used for dental infections and toothaches due to its analgesic and antimicrobial properties. It can be applied topically to the affected area for temporary relief. However, it's essential to consult a dentist for proper evaluation and treatment of dental infections.

Digestive tract infections: Ginger, garlic, and oregano oil can be beneficial for digestive tract infections, including bacterial and parasitic infections.

Ear infections: Mullein oil (Verbascum spp.) is a traditional remedy used for ear infections. It is believed to have anti-inflammatory and antimicrobial properties and may be used topically in the ear canal to help relieve pain and support the healing process. However, it's important to consult a healthcare professional for proper diagnosis and treatment of ear infections.

Eye infections: Eyebright (Euphrasia officinalis) is an herb commonly used for eye infections, such as conjunctivitis (pink eye). It is believed to have anti-inflammatory and antimicrobial properties and can be used as an eyewash or in the form of eye drops.

Fungal infections: Certain herbs like tea tree oil, oregano oil, garlic, and pau d'arco are known for their antifungal properties. They may be used topically or orally to help address fungal infections like athlete's foot, nail fungus, or candidiasis (yeast infections).

Gastrointestinal infections: Certain herbs like peppermint (Mentha piperita), chamomile (Matricaria chamomilla), and fennel (Foeniculum vulgare) are often used to relieve symptoms of gastrointestinal infections such as gastroenteritis, food poisoning, and stomach flu. These herbs can help soothe the digestive system, reduce inflammation, and alleviate symptoms like nausea, vomiting, and diarrhea.

Lyme disease: Certain herbal remedies, such as Japanese knotweed (Polygonum cuspidatum) and cat's claw (Uncaria tomentosa), are sometimes used in the management of Lyme disease, a tick-borne illness. These herbs are believed to have antimicrobial and immune-supporting properties, but their effectiveness and appropriate usage in Lyme disease are still a subject of ongoing research.

Oral infections: Tea tree oil and calendula are sometimes used for oral infections such as gum infections, mouth sores, and thrush.

Parasitic infections: Some herbs, such as wormwood (Artemisia absinthium), black walnut (Juglans nigra), and cloves (Syzygium aromaticum), are believed to have antiparasitic properties and may be used as part of natural protocols for addressing parasitic infections like intestinal parasites or lice. However, it's important to consult with a healthcare professional for proper diagnosis and guidance.

Respiratory infections: Many herbal remedies are used for respiratory infections such as the common cold, sinusitis, bronchitis, and sore throat. Echinacea, garlic, oregano oil, ginger, and eucalyptus are often used to support the immune system and relieve symptoms.

Skin infections: Herbal remedies like calendula, tea tree oil, and lavender oil (Lavandula angustifolia) are commonly used for skin infections, including fungal infections, cuts, wounds, and acne.

Urinary tract infections (UTIs): Certain herbs, such as cranberry (Vaccinium macrocarpon) and uva-ursi (Arctostaphylos uva-ursi), are known to have antimicrobial properties and may provide relief for UTIs.

Vaginal infections: Some herbs, such as tea tree oil, goldenseal, and pau d'arco, may be used topically or as douches to help address certain vaginal infections, including yeast infections and bacterial vaginosis. However, it's important to consult a healthcare professional for accurate diagnosis and appropriate treatment.

Viral infections: Some herbs, such as elderberry, andrographis, and licorice root (Glycyrrhiza glabra), are used to support the immune system and may provide relief for viral infections like the flu and cold sores caused by the herpes simplex virus.

Wound infections: Calendula, lavender oil, and tea tree oil are often used topically for wound care due to their antimicrobial and wound-healing properties. They may help prevent or address mild infections associated with cuts, scrapes, or minor burns.

Yeast infections: Certain herbs like garlic, oregano oil, and pau d'arco (Tabebuia impetiginosa) are believed to have antifungal properties and are sometimes used as complementary remedies for yeast infections.

Medicinal Plants Found in the USA

Providing an exhaustive list of all medicinal herbs found in the United States of America is quite challenging, as the region is vast and encompasses a wide variety of ecosystems and plant species. However, we can offer you a list of some not stated as yet along with a some beneficial notes

Now that we know how to grow most plants and herbs we need to mention the ones that didn't get to make it to the book

Here is a list

1. **Boneset (Eupatorium perfoliatum):** used to reduce fever, increase urine output, cause vomiting, and treat constipation. Boneset is also used to treat influenza, swine flu, acute bronchitis, nasal inflammation, joint pain (rheumatism), fluid retention, dengue fever, and pneumonia; as a stimulant; and to cause sweating.

2. **Elderberry (Sambucus spp.):** The berries and flowers of elderberry are packed with antioxidants and vitamins that may boost your immune system. They could help tame inflammation, lessen stress, and help protect your heart, too. Some experts recommend elderberry to help prevent and ease cold and flu symptoms.

3. **Blue Cohosh (Caulophyllum thalictroides):** the plant "Cohosh" is from the Algonquin Indian word meaning "rough," and it refers to the appearance of the roots. The root is used to make medicine. Blue cohosh is not a safe plant. However, it still is available as a supplement. Sometimes the supplements do not include warnings. It is used for stimulating the uterus and starting labor; starting menstruation; stopping muscle spasms; as a laxative; and for treating colic, sore throat, cramps, hiccups, epilepsy, hysterics, inflammation of the uterus, infection of the female organs (pelvic

inflammatory disease), over-growth of uterine tissue (endometriosis), and joint conditions.

4. **Butterfly Weed (Asclepias tuberosa):** The root of this plant has been used traditionally in Native American medicine. It has been used as a diaphoretic, expectorant, and emetic. It has also been used for lung conditions, such as bronchitis and asthma.

5. **Gravel Root (Eupatorium purpureum):** Also known as Joe-Pye Weed, this herb has been used traditionally as a diuretic and urinary tonic. It has been used to alleviate kidney stones, urinary tract infections, and other urinary system issues.

6. **Lobelia (Lobelia inflata):** has a long history of use as an herbal remedy for respiratory conditions such as asthma, bronchitis, pneumonia, mucus and cough. Historically, Native Americans smoked lobelia as a treatment for asthma.

7. **Oregon Grape (Mahonia spp.):** Oregon grape (Mahonia aquifolium) is a flowering herb that has been used for centuries in traditional Chinese medicine to treat numerous conditions, including psoriasis, stomach issues, heartburn, and low mood.

8. **Osha (Ligusticum porteri):** the root is considered an immune booster and aid for coughs, pneumonia, colds, bronchitis, and the flu. It's also used to relieve indigestion, lung diseases, body aches, and sore throats

9. **Partridgeberry (Mitchella repens):** This herb is used in traditional Native American medicine. It has astringent properties and has been used to support female reproductive health, ease childbirth, and alleviate menstrual discomfort.

10. **Passionflower (Passiflora incarnata):** a climbing vine with white and purple flowers. The chemicals in passion flower have calming effects. Passion flower is native to the southeastern United States and Central and South America. It's been traditionally used to help with sleep. People use passion flower for anxiety, including anxiety before surgery. Some people also take passion flower for insomnia, stress, ADHD, pain, and many other conditions. But there is no good scientific evidence to support these uses. In some foods and beverages, passion flower is added for flavoring.

11. **Prickly Pear Cactus (Opuntia spp.):** Is used for type 2 diabetes, high cholesterol, obesity, alcohol hangover, colitis, diarrhea, and benign prostatic hypertrophy (BPH). It is also used to fight viral infections. In foods, the prickly pear juice is used in jellies and candies.

12. **Rattlesnake Master (Eryngium yuccifolium):** Traditionally used by Native American tribes, this herb has diuretic and diaphoretic properties. It has been used to treat snakebites, promote sweating, and as a urinary tonic.

13. **Saw Palmetto (Serenoa repens):** may help increase testosterone levels, improve prostate health, reduce inflammation, prevent hair loss, and enhance urinary tract function

14. **Sassafras (Sassafras albidum):** Had many medicinal uses as a tea to purify blood and heal ailments including skin diseases, rheumatism, venereal disease, and ague. The roots and berries made a tea to treat nausea, fevers, fatigue, gas pains, menstrual pains, and syphilis. It may also reduce inflammation, act as a diuretic, and help treat leishmaniasis, a parasitic infection.** However, other studies have found that safrole, a compound in sassafras oil, may promote cancer growth. Thus, the FDA has banned its use as a food additive**.

15. **Slippery Elm (Ulmus rubra):** This has been used as healing salves for wounds, boils, ulcers, burns, and skin inflammation. It was also taken orally to relieve coughs, sore throats, diarrhea, and stomach problems. Slippery elm contains mucilage, a substance that becomes a slick gel when mixed with water.

16. **Stoneroot (Collinsonia canadensis):** Stoneroot has been traditionally used for its astringent and diuretic properties. It has been used to treat digestive disorders, hemorrhoids, and urinary conditions.

17. **New Jersey Tea (Ceanothus americanus):** The roots of this plant have been used traditionally as a stimulant and diuretic. It has also been used as a remedy for colds, fevers, and urinary tract conditions.

18. **Usnea (Usnea spp.):** rich in polyphenols, a type of antioxidant that helps fight cell damage caused by unstable compounds known as free radicals. In turn, this antioxidant activity may safeguard against various diseases, including cancer.

19. **Wild Bergamot (Monarda fistulosa):** The Tewa dried the plant and ground it into a powder that was rubbed over the head to cure headaches, over the body to cure fever, and as a remedy for sore eyes and colds. Early white settlers used it as a diaphoretic and carminative, and occasionally employed it for the relief of flatulent colic, nausea and vomiting.

20. **Yarrow (Achillea millefolium):** is a plant that grows throughout the world. The above ground parts are used to make medicine. Yarrow contains chemicals that might

help to stop stomach cramps and fight infections. People commonly use yarrow for eczema, irritable bowel syndrome (IBS), wound healing, and many other conditions, but there is no good scientific evidence to support these uses. Yarrow is sometimes called bloodwort. Don't confuse this with Bloodroot.

This list provides a starting point, but it is by no means exhaustive. There are numerous other medicinal herbs native to the United States, each with its own unique properties and traditional uses. It's important to note that while these herbs have a history of traditional use, it is advisable to consult with a qualified healthcare professional or herbalist for personalized guidance on their safe and effective use. Additionally, proper identification and responsible harvesting practices are essential to preserve wild populations and ecosystems.

Medicinal Plants Specifically for Men

There are several herbs that have been traditionally used to support men's health and well-being. While it's important to consult with a healthcare professional before starting any herbal regimen, here are some herbs that are commonly considered beneficial for men:

Ashwagandha (Withania somnifera): is an adaptogenic herb that has been used in traditional Ayurvedic medicine for centuries and has been traditionally used to support male reproductive health. Some studies suggest that ashwagandha may help increase testosterone levels, improve sperm quality, and enhance fertility. It may also support overall sexual health and performance. Ashwagandha is also considered an adaptogenic herb, which means it helps the body adapt to stress and boosts energy levels. It may improve physical performance, endurance, and stamina, making it beneficial for men who engage in sports or physically demanding activities. Ashwagandha has also been studied for its potential benefits in promoting muscle strength and recovery. It may help increase muscle mass, improve muscle recovery after exercise, and enhance athletic performance.

Cordyceps (Ophiocordyceps sinensis): Also known as the "Chinese caterpillar fungus," the cordyceps mushroom is most frequently found in powder form. This is known for aiding testosterone Levels: Some research suggests that it may help support healthy testosterone levels in men. Testosterone is an important hormone for men's reproductive health, muscle mass, bone density, and overall well-being. As well as your sexual Health: Cordyceps has been used to support male sexual health and enhance libido. It is believed to improve erectile function, increase sperm count and motility, and promote overall sexual vitality.

Hawthorn (Crataegus spp.) is an herb that has been used in traditional medicine for centuries known for heart health: Hawthorn is commonly used to support cardiovascular health. It may help improve blood flow, promote healthy circulation, and support heart function. Maintaining good cardiovascular health is important for overall well-being and can benefit men by supporting optimal blood supply to organs and tissues.

Horny Goat Weed (Epimedium): This herb is commonly used to support male sexual health and address conditions like erectile dysfunction and low libido. This herb is commonly used in traditional Chinese medicine to support sexual health and address erectile dysfunction.

Ginkgo (Ginkgo biloba): known for its cognitive-enhancing properties, supporting memory, focus, and overall brain health. It is also traditionally used to support sexual health and address issues such as erectile dysfunction (ED). It is believed to enhance blood flow to the genital area, increase nitric oxide production, and support overall sexual function

Ginseng (Panax Ginseng): Also known as Korean or Asian ginseng, Panax ginseng is used to support stamina, energy, and overall male vitality. It has been used in traditional medicine to address issues like erectile dysfunction and fatigue.

Linden (Tilia cordata): known for its calming properties and is often used to promote relaxation and relieve stress and anxiety. This can be beneficial for men who experience stress-related health issues or seek support for overall well-being.

Maca (Lepidium meyenii): Maca root is known for its energizing properties, and it has been used to support male sexual health, enhance libido, and improve stamina and endurance and hormonal balance.

Pumpkin seeds(Curcubita pepo): also known as pepitas, offer various health benefits and are considered beneficial for men. Here are some reasons why pumpkin seeds are good for men's health: Pumpkin seeds have been associated with supporting prostate health. They are particularly rich in zinc, which is essential for prostate function and reproductive health in men. Adequate zinc levels may help maintain a healthy prostate gland. Pumpkin seeds also contain compounds like zinc and magnesium, which are associated with supporting healthy testosterone levels. Adequate testosterone levels are important for men's reproductive health, libido, and overall well-being.

Saw Palmetto (Serenoa repens): Saw palmetto is often used to support prostate health and alleviate symptoms associated with benign prostatic hyperplasia (BPH), such as frequent urination and difficulty in emptying the bladder.

Skullcap (Scutellaria lateriflora) is an herb that has been used in traditional herbal medicine for its calming and relaxing properties known to support mood and emotional balance.

Tribulus Terrestris: This herb is believed to support male reproductive health by increasing testosterone levels, improving libido, and enhancing fertility.

Turmeric (Curcuma longa) is a vibrant yellow spice that has been used for centuries in traditional Ayurvedic and Chinese medicine. It contains a compound called curcumin, which is believed to be responsible for many of its health benefits. has been traditionally used to support joint health and alleviate symptoms of arthritis. Its anti-inflammatory properties may help reduce joint pain and improve mobility, making it beneficial for men who experience joint discomfort. Also there are studies suggesting that turmeric may have neuroprotective properties and support cognitive function. This may benefit men's brain health and help maintain mental sharpness and clarity.

Yohimbe (Pausinystalia yohimbe): Yohimbe bark extract is sometimes used to support sexual health and treat erectile dysfunction. However, it's important to note that yohimbe can have significant side effects and interactions with certain medications, so caution is advised.

Medicinal Plants Specifically for Women

There are many herbs that are beneficial for women's health. Here are some examples:

Ashwagandha (Withania somnifera): is a versatile herb used in traditional Ayurvedic medicine. Its adaptogenic properties make it a popular choice among those looking to support their body's natural stress response. Ashwagandha root is also known for its ability to support healthy energy levels, stamina, and cognitive function.*

Ashwagandha may help support healthy thyroid function by balancing TSH levels and improving T4 levels. Additionally, it may help support a healthy immune system by promoting healthy levels of white blood cells.

One of the most notable benefits of Ashwagandha is its ability to support healthy cortisol levels. Cortisol is a hormone that plays a key role in the body's stress response, and when cortisol levels are chronically high, it can lead to negative health effects. Ashwagandha may help to support a healthy cortisol response, which can help to soothe the effects of stress and promote feelings of relaxation.

Black Cohosh (Actaea racemosa): is a plant native to North America and is well-known for supporting a healthy female reproductive system often used to alleviate symptoms of menopause, such as hot flashes and night sweats. Its small, feathery, white flowers make it easily recognizable. Modern herbal preparations often standardize triterpene glycosides, the active constituents of the root. These compounds may be responsible for the herb's effects on the female reproductive system. Herbalists and natural health practitioners have utilized Black Cohosh for its various health benefits. Black Cohosh as a natural remedy has been used since the 1800s to reduce premenstrual syndrome (PMS) symptoms and alleviate menopausal symptoms like hot flashes, night sweats, and mood swings.

Chamomile (Matricaria chamomilla): This herb is often used to ease anxiety, promote relaxation, and support sleep, which can be beneficial for women dealing with stress-related health issues.

Chaste tree berry(Vitex agnus-castus): This herb is often used to support hormonal balance, ease menstrual cramps, and reduce symptoms of premenstrual syndrome (PMS).

Milk thistle: This herb is often used to support liver health and balance hormones, which can be beneficial for women dealing with hormone-related health issues.

Dong Quai (Angelica sinensis): also known as "female ginseng," is an herb used in Traditional Chinese medicine for centuries to support women's health. It is particularly known for supporting healthy menstrual cycles and soothing menopausal symptoms. It is rich in compounds called coumarins, which may support healthy blood circulation and relaxed muscles, making it a popular choice for those looking to soothe the effects of menstrual cramps and support healthy blood flow during menstruation. 9 Dong Quai is typically consumed as a tea, tincture, or capsule.

Evening primrose: (Oenothera biennis): This herb is often used to alleviate symptoms of PMS, as well as support skin health and reduce inflammation.

Fenugreek (Trigonella foenum-graecum): is a plant indigenous to the Mediterranean but is now widely cultivated worldwide. Interestingly, the Latin name for Fenugreek (Trigonella foenum-graecum) means "Greek hay" because the plant was a nutritious addition to cattle feed due to its high nutrient content. People have enjoyed using Fenugreek seeds in traditional medicine and cuisine for centuries. The seeds have a distinct smell, often described as having a faintly sweet aroma, like maple syrup. This unique smell has made Fenugreek seeds a popular ingredient in maple-flavored foods, such as baked goods and syrups. The seeds contain soluble fiber that may help support healthy cholesterol absorption in the bloodstream. One of the most well-known uses of Fenugreek is to support the optimal production of breast milk in nursing mothers. This is due to compounds in the seeds that support milk production, including phytoestrogens and galactagogues. While this is the traditional use of Fenugreek, it is always best to consult a healthcare provider before using it to support lactation.

Ginseng (Panax ginseng): is a perennial herb that may support healthy libido and fertility in women. Ginseng may also support healthy menstrual cycles. Ginseng supplements are an easy and convenient way to add the benefits of this herb to your daily routine. Ginseng is available in many forms, including supplements, teas, and extracts. It has a slightly bitter taste, which can be masked by adding it to food or drinks. Ginseng is also known for its adaptogenic properties, meaning it helps the body better cope with feelings of stress and supports healthy immune function.

Lavender: This herb is often used to promote relaxation and reduce anxiety, and can be especially beneficial for women dealing with menstrual-related anxiety or insomnia.

Lemon balm: This herb is often used to promote relaxation, reduce anxiety, and support sleep, and can be beneficial for women dealing with stress-related health issues.

Maca (Lepidium meyenii): is a knobby root vegetable that resembles a turnip, a relative of this native Peruvian plant. This hardy adaptogenic herb grows best in the harsh environment of the high Andes, where the Inca warriors used it as a caffeine-free performance enhancer. Maca root may help soothe the effects of vaginal dryness and support healthy energy, stamina, and libido in women. Traditional medicine has used maca root for centuries, particularly in the Andean region, to soothe various health issues. Recent research has shown that it may support natural fertility by helping to maintain normal reproductive hormone levels. In women, Maca may support healthy levels of luteinizing hormone (LH), follicle-stimulating hormone (FSH), and estrogen, which are important for healthy reproductive function. It has a delicious, somewhat nutty taste, and Maca Powder, the powdered form of this herb, can be added to smoothies, juice, or oatmeal, making it a convenient way to add its nutritional benefits to your diet. In addition, there are also Maca root pills.

Passionflower: This herb is often used to promote relaxation and reduce anxiety, and can be beneficial for women dealing with menstrual-related anxiety or insomnia.

Raspberry Leaf

Supports women's reproductive health and hormone balance. Raspberry Leaf (Rubus idaeus) is a perennial shrub that also grows natively in Europe and Asia. This herb is a rich source of vitamins and minerals, including vitamins C and E, calcium, and magnesium, which are essential for healthy reproductive function.Raspberry Leaf is also known for its ability to support a strong and toned uterus, which may help women during childbirth. Midwives often recommend Raspberry Leaf to support normal labor and delivery, minimize the need for interventions during childbirth, and support a healthy recovery after giving birth. Controlled trials are needed to verify these claims further. Raspberry Leaf has a slightly sweet and earthy flavor, and it can be brewed as tea or added to smoothies. It is also available in supplement form, including capsules and tinctures

Red Clover (Trifolium pratense): is a highly versatile and nutritious herb that has long supported women's health. It is an excellent choice for supporting women's health during menopause. It is a rich source of naturally occurring phytoestrogens that help support healthy estrogen levels in women to support uterine and ovarian health. Red Clover also encourages detoxification, promotes healthy skin, and supports the body's lymphatic functions. Native to North America, Red Clover has since spread across Europe and into the Far East and has a rich history of use in Russian and Chinese herbalism. Red Clover's highly nutritious properties continue to make it a popular food for grazing livestock. Its wide range of benefits makes it a valuable addition to any natural health routine.

Shatavari (Asparagus racemosus): is an herb commonly used in Ayurvedic medicine to support female reproductive health, including healthy menstruation and lactation, and may also support healthy libido and fertility. It's also a natural aphrodisiac that may help to support sexual function and desire in women and soothe the effects of vaginal dryness.

Ayurvedic medicine considers it a "Rasayana" or rejuvenating herb and may help the female reproductive system by promoting healthy menstrual cycles and supporting fertility.

St. John's wort: This herb is often used to alleviate symptoms of mild depression and anxiety, which can be especially beneficial for women experiencing mood swings related to their menstrual cycle or menopause.

Vitex (Vitex agnus-castus) is also called Chaste Tree. Its Latin name means "chaste lamb," and in ancient times, its leaves were strewn at the feet of clergy to keep them as the plant's name implies!

Healthy hormone levels are necessary for physical and emotional well-being.* Vitex has been used since the time of Hippocrates to support gynecological health, particularly for the changing seasons and cycles of life.* Used traditionally to support healthy and regular menstrual cycles, soothe PMS symptoms, and support hormone production and balance. 4 This herb's berries promote a healthy mind and body throughout the menstrual cycle and during the transition into menopause.

Endangered Medicinal Plants:
(Found in North America)

There are many herbs that are endangered due to habitat destruction, over-harvesting, climate change, and other environmental factors. Here are some examples of endangered herbs:

American ginseng (Panax quinquefolius): This herb is native to North America and has been over-harvested for its medicinal properties. It is now considered endangered in the wild and is heavily regulated.

Goldenseal (Hydrastis canadensis): This herb is also native to North America and has been over-harvested for its medicinal properties. It is now listed as endangered in several states. Bearberry (Arctostaphylos uva-ursi)

Black cohosh (Actaea racemosa):

Blue cohosh (Caulophyllum thalictroides)

Bloodroot (Sanguinaria canadensis)

Goldenseal (Hydrastis canadensis)

Hoodia (Hoodia gordonii):

Osha root (Ligusticum porteri):

Rattlesnake master (Eryngium yuccifolium)

Sanicle (Sanicula spp.)

Slippery elm (Ulmus rubra)

Trillium (Trillium spp.)

Wild yam (Dioscorea villosa)

Virginia snakeroot (Aristolochia serpentaria)

Wild ginger (Asarum canadense)

Yerba mansa (Anemopsis californica)

It is important to be aware of the endangered status of these herbs and to practice sustainable harvesting methods or purchase them from reputable sources that do so in order to help protect these important plant species

About Authors

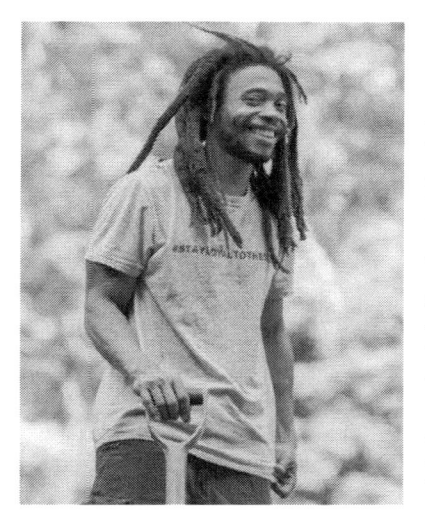

Shawn Joseph: Starting his gardening journey at the young age of 7 Shawn developed his love and passion for all things plants very early. Over the years he sharpened his skills growing a variety of plants in many different ways and learned how they interact with each other & the surrounding environment. This curiosity of plant propagation continued as he pursued and obtained his degree in horticulture. As a horticulturist Shawn currently spends his days farming and volunteering his time to help others learn the ways of organic gardening and providing healthy options all while gaining patience & appreciation for the natural world we live in.

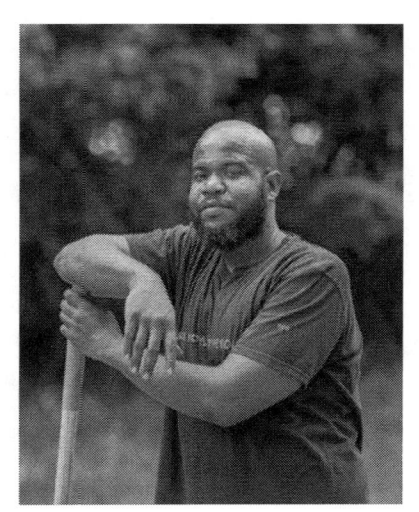

Richard Myers;

Being born on an island where everyone is dependent on nature, Richard fell in love with plants at a young age. He was able to understand the importance of having one's own crops, whether it was to feed the family, donate, or sell. Seeking an education that would match his love for plants led him towards Horticulture (The art and science of plants) and he hasn't turned back since.

Made in the USA
Middletown, DE
08 February 2024